CRYSTALS FOR HEALING

Your Beginners Guide to Crystals and Healing Stones

(The Ultimate Beginner's Guide to Crystals and Their Uses)

Elvis Etheridge

Published by Harry Barnes

Elvis Etheridge

All Rights Reserved

Crystals for Healing: Your Beginners Guide to Crystals and Healing Stones (The Ultimate Beginner's Guide to Crystals and Their Uses)

ISBN 978-1-7751430-0-0

All rights reserved. No part of this guide may be reproduced in any form without permission in writing from the publisher except in the case of brief quotations embodied in critical articles or reviews.

Legal & Disclaimer

The information contained in this book is not designed to replace or take the place of any form of medicine or professional medical advice. The information in this book has been provided for educational and entertainment purposes only.

The information contained in this book has been compiled from sources deemed reliable, and it is accurate to the best of the Author's knowledge; however, the Author cannot guarantee its accuracy and validity and cannot be held liable for any errors or omissions. Changes are periodically made to this book. You must consult your doctor or get professional medical advice before using any of the suggested remedies, techniques, or information in this book.

Upon using the information contained in this book, you agree to hold harmless the Author from and against any damages, costs, and expenses, including any legal fees potentially resulting from the application of any of the information provided by this guide. This disclaimer applies to any damages or injury caused by the use and application, whether directly or indirectly, of any advice or information presented, whether for breach of contract, tort, negligence, personal injury, criminal intent, or under any other cause of action.

You agree to accept all risks of using the information presented inside this book. You need to consult a professional medical practitioner in order to ensure you are both able and healthy enough to participate in this program.

Table of Contents

INTRODUCTION 1

CHAPTER 1: HEALING BLINGS 3

CHAPTER 2: WHAT IS CRYSTAL HEALING? 12

CHAPTER 3: UNDERSTAND CRYSTAL HEALING 16

CHAPTER 4: WHAT IS A CRYSTAL AND HOW DOES IT FORM 21

CHAPTER 5: HISTORY OF CRYSTALS AND CRYSTAL HEALING 30

CHAPTER 6: THE PRACTICAL WAYS TO USE HEALING CRYSTALS FOR PHYSICAL, MENTAL, EMOTIONAL AND SPIRITUAL HEALING 52

CHAPTER 7: OVERVIEW ON CRYSTAL THERAPY 63

CHAPTER 8: USING CRYSTALS FOR HEALING 103

CHAPTER 9: HOW CAN I IMPROVE MY LIFE WITH CRYSTALS? 118

CHAPTER 10: INDIVIDUAL GEMSTONES & CRYSTALS 143

CONCLUSION 181

Introduction

Whether to adorn the crowns of powerful kings and queens, to give power to a mage's staff, or to channel energy when building and casting spells, crystals have always been associated with magic, power, and mysterious mystic forces. Although not as exaggerated as in fantasy books and games, crystals do carry power with them, as well as deep symbolism that goes back to the dawn of time. There is a whole world to discover when it comes to crystals, and it can be daunting and a little scary to explore, especially if you don't know where to start. That is precisely what this book is for. Whether you're a fresh new explorer carefully testing the waters for the first time or an experienced spelunker who's been diving in and out of the hidden nooks and crannies of the crystal world for years, this book will help you understand crystals a bit better.

Not only will this book give an explanation on how crystals work, where they come from, what they look like, and what they do, but it will also show you how you can use crystals to improve your own life from aligning chakras and boosting the effects of meditation to using crystals in simple ways to alleviate stress and depression and improving almost all aspects of your everyday life.

To take it a step further, this book will help guide you in building your own personal crystal collection and one that works best for you, and it will teach you how to care for and maintain your collection, as well as how to best use it to its full potential.

Furthermore, you will be reading a list of the most prominent and important crystals with clear descriptions, where they come from, and how they can be used, making it easy to identify your crystals.

Chapter 1: Healing Blings

Think about the last time that you got infected with a simple sickness, a headache, perhaps. What sort of medicine did you take? Did you go to the hospital to see a doctor? What kind of medical procedures did you go through? Did you ever consider taking alternative medicine? If your answer to this last question is a big definite "no", then it is a sign that you are definitely dependent on synthetic drugs and medications. In fact, it is not only you who is. Most of us are just like you. We all live in a society wherein it is the norm to always quickly resort to pills and tablets whenever we have a simple cold or a cough or whenever we feel anxious or lonely. We were so used to the idea of popping a pill whenever we have an illness or a disease.

See, ever since the use of synthetic medical cures which birthed out of the laboratories of pharmaceutical companies became popular as well as the medical procedures that were introduced by doctors became the norms in healing and in relieving pain, illness and discomfort, we already forgot about the existence, importance and the benefits of alternative medicines and natural healing techniques. We have been blinded by the technicalities of medical procedures and medicines that we are already willing to take them and go through them even though we are aware that most of these medicines and procedures have negative side effects and can cause complications to our bodies, as well as to the natural niche of the systems of the Earth. We are so blinded by these products that we have come to the point of advertising and patronizing the same products that trash the environment and make us even more terrible.

We already forgot about the fact that there are healing procedures that our ancestors used during their time and that are effective, safe and most importantly, free or at least, does not cost that much of a fortune. Because of this, alternative medicine and alternative healing procedures were almost threatened to disappear.

As an answer to the fact that medical products produced by major pharmaceutical companies can be bad for our health instead of being good, some people have turned back to the natural ways of healing. Alternative medicine is a booming business during this zeitgeist and a lot of people are now patronizing these herbal products and preferring them over the synthetic cures that come out from medical laboratories.

The main premise that these alternative products hold is the natural healing effects of nature. The advocates of natural healing products argue that most of the ingredients that are in the synthetic drugs that pharmaceuticals produce can already be found in the environment through the existence of plants and minerals. That is why it is irrelevant to make synthetic counterparts to the cures that are already within our reach. During this age, people are more open to the idea of using natural medicines because they are now knowledgeable about the side effects of synthetic drugs and the harmful effects that the production of these drugs can cause to the environment. Buyers are more skeptical and more meticulous when it comes to the ingredients and the effects of the products that they ingest.

And so, numerous herbal products spread like wildfire in the market and hundreds and thousands of supplies are selling like they are hot cakes. Alternative healing procedures such as massage therapies, yoga schools, meditation centers and nature based healing are becoming more popular to the people. Asian ways of curing such as acupuncture have also made their way towards piquing the interest of consumers all over the globe.

But little do we know, there is another way of healing that most of us do not have or have little awareness about. In fact, the main tool that this healing technique uses is just commonly used as ornaments in art, or as jewelry and blings, or as embellishments to dresses and other types of clothing. This natural healing procedure is called **crystal healing.** What is crystal healing, you ask? Well, crystal healing is a kind of alternative healing procedure or therapy that involves crystals (Yes. I am talking about the same crystals that are in your earrings or the ones that you wear as jewelry right now.) as well as other stones in order to aid feelings of pain and discomfort brought about by diseases and illnesses. This type of alternative medical procedure is not invasive and is holistic. This means you will not be required to ingest anything or take something in order for you to be cured. Also, not only one component of your body will be target but as well the other organs and parts that make your body a whole.

Crystal healing involves harmonizing the mind, spirit, body and the feelings and emotions in order to gain tranquility, to alleviate the feelings of stress and negativity, to make our well-being more positive and to make our bodily system a bit more incorporated.

According to history and ancient artifacts and proofs, the practice of crystal healing has been around for more or less 6,000 years already. The place where it actually came from, however, remains unknown and uncertain. Although this is the case, there are accounts that traced the roots of crystal healing all the way back from the time of the Sumerians in the ancient fertile lands of Mesopotamia. There has also been a proof that the first people who used crystals in order to ward off negative spirits and diseases were the Egyptians of Ancient Egypt. It has been said that Egyptians adorned themselves in turquoise, lapis lazuli, carnelian and other precious crystals and stones solely for this purpose.

Now, crystal healing is already used as an alternative medicine that people prefer over synthetic drugs in order to feel relief from common diseases and ailments.

Although there has been testimonials and personal accounts of relief reaped out from doing this alternative healing procedure, a lot of medical practitioners are still skeptical about this healing technique. As there is a resistance to herbal medicine from the medical and scientific experts, there is also a resistance in practicing crystal healing to cure people. This is because of the argument that the principles used in crystal healing are not really scientific. Doctors and scientists only identify it as a pseudoscience and cannot be entirely reliable when it comes to healing a person from his or her sickness. This is mainly because they found no evidential information about a flowing energy form of some sort that causes sickness or ailment. Some even say this is just a form of sorcery or magic or even an act of darkness because energies and chakras are involved, both of which by the way, are not visible to the naked eye. Maybe that is also a reason why crystal healing is not accepted in the medical world. It is because this form of healing technique involves something that cannot be seen and for us, something that cannot be seen by our own two eyes is not really real and legitimate.

However, this book aims to enthuse and encourage you to explore the art of crystal healing. It aims to open your eyes to its possibility and hope that you will be open minded to its possibility. It will teach you what crystal healing is all about and how you can unleash the powers of crystals to help you ward off your sickness and symptoms and that of others. It will also teach you and make you understand its basic concepts and ideas. Knowing about this procedure is just the first step into gaining mastery and success in this craft. You will still have a lot to learn and the following chapter will help you learn all of those things.

Chapter 2: What Is Crystal Healing?

Crystal healing is an alternative medicine technique that utilizes stones and crystals to restore internal balance, relieve stress, and increase a person's energy. This is commonly done by allowing the practitioner to place crystals on various parts of your body, specifically on your chakras. Another way is to surround the person's body with crystals in order to create an energy grid, which will envelop you in healing energy.

Contrary to what most people may believe in, the use of precious stone for healing is not some new-age fad. The use of healing crystals actually dates back to ancient civilizations. Ancient Egyptians, for instance, have been known to use the rose quartz to help in beautification and the amethyst was worn by envoys to protect them in their travels. The knowledge of crystal healing has been passed down throughout the eras, thus, making it a time-tested tradition that defies differences in culture and religion.

Are crystals magical then?

Some people would like to think so. However, for skeptics, there is a more sensible explanation as to how crystals are able to affect one's energy balance and state of health. What most people fail to realize is that crystals are living beings—complete with protons, neutrons, and electrons, all cooperating to maintain the arrangement of the stone's sacred geometry. They are a part of nature and as such, each precious stone consists of its own energy. They produce resonance in both the physical and the spiritual plane. They emit vibrations that in turn, affect your own energy vibrations. While the energy from some stones can help increase your levels of vitality, the energy in others may provide a calming effect. In the end, it is all a matter of balance and it is up to you to use these crystals and their energies to suit your current needs.

How do these crystals work?

To fully grasp the healing mechanism of precious stones, it is necessary to accept the belief that everything in and of this universe has the potential to heal. Our whole body system is simply energy that manifests in different densities and patterns. Notice that despite our diversity, all natural beings are constructed in pretty much the same manner—from the circulation of blood in our veins to the circulation of air within our lungs, each is like its own miniature ecosystem. As long as these energy patterns maintain their balance, we are able to enjoy a state of wellbeing. However, once these patterns are disturbed, we experience discomfort and disease. Thankfully, nature has a way of healing itself. And even as we continue to interfere with this harmony through our habits and behavior, it is possible for us to restore this harmony by making use of anything which contains inherent balance. Enter, healing crystals. That said, in order for this healing technique to work, one must become utterly receptive. Healing stones possess the energy of the earth within them. When you allow them to come in contact with your body, you allow yourself to come in contact with the earth's vitality.

Chapter 3: Understand Crystal Healing

It is believed that crystal healing dates back as far back as 6000 years to the time of the Sumerians in Mesopotamia. It is also believed that the ancient Egyptians were some of the first to practice crystal healing.

Today, crystal healing is predominantly based on traditional concepts of Asian cultures, where some of the people believed in the energy of life. The chakras, a part of modern healing with crystals, also date back to traditional Asian cultures through Buddhism and Hinduism. It is said to connect the physical and supernatural elements of the body.

It is believed that crystal healing is a natural form of medicine that receives its powers through different stones to which several properties are assigned. During a normal session, a healer may place stones in the body in different areas or may suggest that you use certain stones to repel disease or absorb positive energy. Because each stone has a different power, it is believed that using these stones and crystals can restore balance and stability to the energy system of the body, allowing natural healing processes to take place.

Learn the Different Chakras.

There are so many different crystals, so it would be difficult to memorize them but there are only seven chakras and it can be useful to learn them so that you are aware of the imbalances you might experience in your body.

The crown chakra: located at the top of your head, this chakra helps to connect with your spiritual self, promotes imagination, inspiration and positive thinking.

The third eye chakra: situated just above the eyebrows, this chakra balances the glands of the endocrine system and therefore, affects vision, intuition, psychic abilities, concentration, self-knowledge and insight.

The throat chakra: located in the throat, this chakra helps you connect with the world around you, affecting communication, self-expression and sound.

The heart chakra: situated in the center of the chest, this chakra deals with emotions and therefore, helps create compassion, love, understanding, sharing and forgiveness.

The solar plexus chakra: situated between the navel and the base of the ribcage, this chakra creates confidence, humor, personal power, authority, laughter and warmth and also helps you shape your identity and personality.

The sacral bone chakra: located between the navel and the pubic bone, this chakra promotes physical strength, vitality and also generates new ideas, creativity, passion, endurance and sexual energy.

The perineum chakra: located at the base of the spine, this chakra promotes physical survival, vitality, stability, patience and courage.

It is a Pseudoscience

While it is a traditional practice, many doctors and modern scientists do not support crystal healing as an appropriate form of medicine because there are no arbitrated articles that prove their abilities. Often, when undergoing crystal therapy, participants experience positive feelings due to this placebo effect.

While it is okay to try crystal therapy, if you or someone you know suffers from a dangerous or serious illness, you should consider visiting a doctor instead of a healer. Crystal therapy is an effective form of therapeutic medicine if you seek to calm your mind and possibly relieve depression.

Become a Healer with Crystals

To practice crystal therapy, many offices require a certification or license through a university or school that practices natural medicinal techniques. Crystal therapy is no different than massages or physical exercise in the sense that therapists ultimately help their patients experience relaxation and stress relief.

Chapter 4: **What Is A Crystal And How Does It Form**

Crystals are beautiful rock formations that have astounded people for thousands of years. They're used in many ways, not only as decorations. Years ago, radios were projected to make use of crystals to convey radio waves. Some instruments, such as quartz watches, still use crystals to this day. They have always been seen as something of value and are often put inside parts of jewelry with diamonds or other jewels. Most of the crystals are now human-made in laboratories. They are highly uncommon to be found on Earth.

What Are Crystals?

Crystals are nothing more than a fixed set of molecules or atoms. Crystals come in many different shapes and sizes and each has different features. What they're produced of determines how it's going to be formed. Some shells can be produced of salt— they create cubed crystals. Many are composed from other elements and shape entirely different forms. Examples of these are diamonds or rubies. There are some components that could produce more than one form. When the carbon element is in the form of a diamond, it can be used to cut gemstones, but we use it on a daily basis, in different manners. The most important way we use it is to deliver electricity to our homes and companies.

How Crystals Are Formed

If you would like to understand how crystals are formed, you can experiment in your own kitchen and see crystals forming with your own eyes. This can be achieved by placing a tiny quantity of table salt in some standard tap water, waiting for 24 hours and you'll see some beautiful cubed structures. This occurs because water evaporates, which allows the atoms that compose the salt (mineral) and water to grow nearer together. Eventually they're going to create a good little uniform bunch of atoms. The more they can come together, the more the structure becomes noticeable to the naked eye. Scientists can determine what mineral they're looking at by the way crystals are formed.

Not all the crystals are formed in the water. Many are crystallized in carbon. However, all crystals shape the same manner; atoms come together and become a group of uniforms. The process could take from a few days to maybe a thousand years. Natural crystals coming from Earth are the same thing. These crystals were formed in the crust of the Earth over a million years ago. They happen when the liquid in the earth is consolidated and the temperature chills. Other crystals shape when the liquid passes through the cracks and disperses the minerals into the cracks.

Interesting Facts on Crystals

Even without realizing, we use or see crystals often - salt, sugar, gemstones and snowflakes. Crystals are valued for their beauty of gemstones and appreciated for being useful in many electronic products. Some individuals also think that crystals have spiritual and healing characteristics. Their organized, repeated models are a marvel of nature and chemistry.

Types of Crystals

Crystals can shape in many forms, from simple cubic constructions to hexagonal or double pyramids to large spires with up to 10 or more sides. Some of them are not symmetrical from one hand to the other. The form of the crystal structure is determined by its chemical components and chemical bonds. Sometimes the crystalline structure shifts to the liquid state and becomes a liquid crystal often used in the present technology.

Common Crystals

Quartz is a crystal that many people understand. It develops in six-sided boxes and can come in a variety of colors, based on the chemical impurities in the column. An amethyst gemstone is a quartz form with chemicals that offer it a wealthy purple color. Table salt is a crystal formed by two chemicals, sodium and chloride, which come together in a cube-shaped crystalline structure. Epsom salts, used for healing, are produced of magnesium and sulfur and form a spicy, crystal-clear shape.

Where Crystals Come From

Natural crystals are dug out of the ground, where the temperature and stress of the earth lead them to form. Many crystals are also produced in laboratories under monitored circumstances for particular reasons.

Uses for Crystals

Quartz crystals have a natural property called piezoelectricity, the capacity to produce an electrical field that makes them very helpful in radio and video machinery. Silicon crystals are used to make chips that power our computers and photovoltaic cells used in solar technology. Crystals are often sliced and polished into jewels used in jewelry. Crystals are often used as ornamental artifacts and focal points for meditation and healing.

Make Your Own Crystals

At home, you can form your crystals. You'll need a heat-resistant glass container, a measuring cup, 1/2 cup of salt, 1 cup of cooking water, a pencil, a paper clip, a cotton cord, a spoon and a paper towel.

Tie the stick to one side of the pencil and the other end of the paper clip. Place your pencil across the bottom of your container. The cable is scarcely supposed to let the paper clip reach the ground. Boil 1 cup of water and add it to the container. Add 1/2 cup of salt to the water, one teaspoon at the moment. Stir in the water for each teaspoon until it dissolves. If you discover some salt in the bottom of the bottle, you can avoid adding more. This implies that the solution is "supersaturated." Put a string and a paper clip in a bottle with a on top and cover with a paper towel. After two days, you'll see a lot of crystals forming along the paper clip and the cord.

How Does a Sugar Crystal Grow?

Place a small quantity of sugar on a surface where is easy to observe it. You will be able to see that it is made of millions of small crystals. Now, if you put the same quantity of sugar in water, what happens is that the small particles disintegrate shortly after the contact. If you want to recrystallize the sugar, you have to choose between the two following methods.

Evaporation Reaction

Sugar molecules are the most stable ones in the crystalline structure. If you leave the solution of sugar submerged in water exposed, the water will evaporate and the solution will become increasingly focused.

As the water molecules vanish, the sugar molecules discover each other and return to the crystals.

Supersaturation and Precipitation

A limited quantity of sugar is dissolved in cold water, but greater temperatures enable the liquid to contain more sugar molecules. The hot liquid is a supersaturated solution. When the temperature is moderate, there is not enough space for the sugar molecules, so they return to a solid-state, translucent structure through a process called precipitation.

Growing Crystals

Crystals are growing and still not alive and they seem to produce order out of nothing. For these purposes, researchers have been excited for thousands of years. Crystals are prevalent and simple to produce, even if they require a little research to comprehend. Producing crystals and studying them is so intriguing that it may not seem like a work project at all.

Chapter 5: History Of Crystals And Crystal Healing

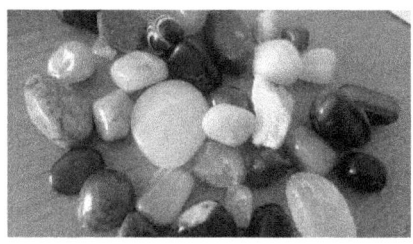

Human beings have always had a mysterious connection and attraction toward crystals and stones since time immemorial as previously explained. Stunning amulets, talismans, and jewelry made of crystals have been unearthed from ancient civilizations that flourished thousands and thousands of years ago.

The history of crystals goes so way back that we have no clear idea to pinpoint a certain period when the use of these beautiful stones became such an integral part of human life. Ivory beads dating back to more than 60,000 years have been excavated in Sungir, Russia. This period is part of the Paleolithic Age when human beings were just about beginning to change from the nomadic hunter-gatherer lifestyle to a life of settled communities.

Jet also seemed to have been a popular stone used during the Paleolithic Age. In Belgium and Switzerland, jet beads, amulets, and jewelry belonging to the Paleolithic Age have been excavated from gravesites dating back to the Paleolithic Age.

The oldest amulets known to human beings were made of Baltic amber, which are believed to be more than 30,000 years old. Amulets made with Baltic amber excavated in Britain have been dated to be older than 10,000 years, which marks the beginning of the Ice Age. The fact that crystals were taken from the Baltic region to Britain illustrates the importance given to stones and amulets even during those ancient times. Malachite mines in Sinai have been in existence from 4000 B.C.

In 355 A.D., the Christian Church banned the use of amulets although crystals and gemstones continued to be popular right through ancient and medieval history. Interestingly, sapphire was a favored and well-liked gemstone in the priestly fraternity as this gem was used to make ecclesiastical rings during the 11th and 12th centuries. In the 11th century, the Bishop of Rennes said that wearing rings made with agate made the wearer increase his favor with God! Another crystal-based symbol used in Christianity was that of carbuncle to represent Christ's sacrifice.

Historical References of Crystals and Gemstones in Ancient Cultures

Ancient Sumerians employed crystals to create magic formulas. Lapis lazuli, carnelian, turquoise, and clear quartz were commonly used by Ancient Egyptians to make jewelry and ornaments. The Egyptians also used these crystals to design burial ornaments, many of which have been unearthed by archeologists. The ancient Mayans believed that the souls of people who lived morally upright and good lives on earth went into crystals.

Turquoise was considered to be a stone that bridged heaven and earth. This belief is held by numerous Native American tribes as well as the people of Tibet. One particular Native American legend says that if you could reach the end of a rainbow and dig up the earth there, you would find turquoise.

Lapis lazuli was believed to be a royal stone in ancient Egypt. It was ground and powdered and rubbed on to the crown of the head because the ancient Egyptians believed that this royal crystal had the power to eliminate all negative energies and other impurities from your body.

It is believed that the Ancient Egyptians and Sumerians used crystals and gemstones mainly for health and protection. Chrysolite was used to purge evil spirits and fight off fears about darkness and night. However, the innovative Egyptians also used crystals to make cosmetics. For example, they used ground and powdered lead ore (galena) and malachite to make kohl, an eye cosmetic used to darken and highlight the shape of the eye.

Malachite also adorned the headdress of Egyptian pharaohs because they believed that this stone helped them to rule and govern wisely. Malachite powder was used to treat vision problems and was also used to help people improve their inner vision. In funerals, green stones were used as they are believed to signify the heart of the dead person. This ritual of using green stones in burials was followed later on in Mexican culture too.

Additionally, an ancient hieroglyphic papyrus believed to belong to 2000 B.C. reveals the use of crystals for medicinal purposes. Other documents dating back to 1500 B.C. also speak of the multiple medicinal benefits of crystals.

Ancient Greeks have a special to crystals for many reasons including:

● Most of the modern-day names of crystals and gemstones originate in the ancient Greek language.

● The Ancient Greeks attributed special properties to the gemstones for healing and protection purposes

Here are some crystal names connected to the Greek language:

● The word 'crystal' itself is Greek for ice. It was believed that clear quartz was nothing but water frozen so deeply that it could not thaw out even in the presence of heat and would remain in solid form forever.

- The word 'amethyst', which is Greek for 'not drunken.' Amethyst was commonly used to prevent drunkenness and as treatments for hangovers.

- 'Hematite' means blood in Greek, and the stone got this name because of the blood-red coloration it took on during the oxidation process. Hematite is iron ore, and iron was a metal the Greeks related to the God of War, Aries. When Greek soldiers went out on battle, they rubbed their bodies with hematite because they believed that iron would make them invulnerable.

Also, Greek sailors wore a number of protective amulets during their voyages.

The Ancient Chinese culture gave prime importance to jade. In fact, some of the Chinese written characters look like jade beads. This gemstone was so much revered in China that many ancient emperors were buried in armor made of jade. Interestingly, jade masks were unearthed when graves from Mexico from around the same time were excavated. In China, wind chimes made of jade were used for protection against evil spirits.

In many Far East nations including China and Japan, quartz was considered to be the heart or the core of dragons. By the way, dragons were believed to have great power, and also symbolically, a dragon represented a wise and highly evolved person.

Both in the cultures of South America and China, jade were considered to have powerful kidney healing powers. In more recent history, the Maoris of New Zealand were known to wear jade pendants, which were passed on for generations through the male lineage. In some parts of New Zealand, green stones like jade are revered for their lucky charm capabilities even today.

An important prehistoric site that reflects the importance of crystals in the history of humankind is the Solar Temple in Newgrange, Ireland. Considered older than the pyramids of Egypt, this site is a passage grave in Ireland's Boyne Valley. It was constructed in such a way that on the day of the Winter Solstice, the sun's rays would stream and be reflected through the 70-foot long entrance, which was originally covered with white quartz, a crystal that symbolizes the White Goddess.

Many ancient Native American tribes used crystals for ceremonial, healing, and protective purposes. Some of these people used crystals for practical purposes as well. For example, the people of the ancient Mexican civilization used pyrite to make mirrors. Obsidian was a crystal highly revered by the Mayans who used it to make ceremonial knives and also to improve their physical as well as inner vision.

Crystals and Gemstones in Religion

Nearly all religions across the world have references to crystals and gemstones in their scriptures and holy books. Crystals are mentioned in numerous places in the Bible, Koran, and multiple other religious books. The Book of Exodus mentions that all birthstones originated from the 'High Priest's Breastplate,' which is the breastplate of Aaron.

According to the Koran, the 4th heaven is made of carbuncle. In Hinduism, the Kalpa tree, a sacred tree used as offerings to the gods, is believed to be made entirely of precious and semi-precious stones. A 7th-century Buddhist text mentions a diamond throne near the Tree of Knowledge under which Lord Buddha meditated. A thousand Kalpa Buddhas are supposed to be reposing on this diamond throne.

In Jainism too, there is a mention of crystals and gemstones. A Jainism scripture, Kalpa Sutra, talks about Harinegamesi, a divine and powerful leader of foot soldiers. This gifted commander captured 14 precious stones, cleansed them of all their negative properties and energies, and retained only the core, unadulterated essence of the stones. Harinegamesi is believed to have used the power of these stones for transformation purposes.

An Indian lapidary (lapidary relates to the polishing and cutting of precious and semi-precious stones) document titled Ratnapariksha Buddhabhatta believed to be from the 6th century Buddhism texts talks about diamond being the king of all gemstones. The Sanskrit word for diamond is 'Vajra' which is the name of the thunderbolt belonging to Indra, the King of Gods, according to Hindu mythology. In Hinduism, diamonds are often connected with thunder.

This lapidary treatise also talks about ruby and many other gemstones and crystals and their powers and properties. The ruby was highly revered by many religions and believed to represent an eternal flame.

The ruby's power is in its ability to protect and preserve the physical and mental health of the wearer.

Crystals during the Renaissance Period

European history is replete with numerous texts and treatises on crystals written from the 11th century until the Renaissance. These texts extol the powers and magical properties of crystals and gemstones including their healing powers in certain diseases. During these times, stones were combined with herbal therapies.

Authors from the Renaissance Period who wrote books and treatises on crystals and gemstones include John Mandeville, Hildegard von Binghen, and Arnoldus Saxo. The books written by these people have references to stones naturally empowered with certain health and protective properties.

There is an interesting historical anecdote about the belief in the power of gemstones. In 1232, a general in the army of King Henry III is believed to have stolen a crystal from the king's treasury, and given it to the King of Wales, an arch enemy of King Henry III. This particular crystal was known for it ability to make the wearer invincible.

It was also believed that crystals were corrupted by Adam, the first man, and sinners who wore gemstones could run the risk of losing all their virtues and good qualities. It was, therefore, imperative to cleanse, sanctify, and clear all crystals of negative energies before wearing them. Cleansing of crystals is a vital part of crystal care even today.

While the power of crystals was accepted by many people during the Renaissance Period, the science-based enquiring and questioning attitude of the society at that time also resulted in raising doubts in the minds of the believers. People wanted a scientific explanation as to how crystals had healing capabilities.

Crystal Healing

So, when did the modern age of crystal healing start? Anselm de Boot is usually credited with the modern scientific explanation for the power of crystals. In 1609, this court physician to Rudolf II of Germany said that the power of crystals (whether good or bad) was the result of good and bad angles within the structure of the crystal.

He stated that the good angels rendered good qualities like healing and protective powers to gemstones, and the bad angles created negative energies in the crystals. He said that the power of crystals was not the effect of anything divine or godly. Anselm de Boot even listed the names of some crystals that were helpful and some that were not helpful, or even, could produce harmful effects on the wearer. All qualities that could not be explained using the bad and good angles were simply brushed of as superstitions.

During the same time, Thomas Nichols wrote a book called 'A Faithful Lapidary,' in which he claimed that all crystals and other inanimate objects did not have any qualities and healing powers as claimed in the past. And so, during the later stages of the Renaissance Period, the use of crystals in healing began to decline, especially in Europe.

Then, in the early 19th century, many interesting experiments were conducted to prove the healing power of crystals and gemstones. People who believed themselves to be clairvoyants expressed that not only were they able to feel the emotional and mental healing powers of the stones but were also able to feel physical sensations like smell and touch.

Crystal Healing in the Modern Times

Today, although crystals are not used in modern western medicines, they continue to hold significance and meaning for numerous ancient cultures around the world. In fact, until the middle of the 20th century, a garnet was worn by soldiers who went out into battle, and jet was worn during funerals and as a sign of mourning.

In a culture that is still prevalent in southwest England, before her wedding, the daughter of the house is expected to wear a moonstone necklace (a symbol of fertility), which is typically like an heirloom passed on for generations in her family. Other tribal cultures that continue to revere crystals and their healing powers even today are:

- In New Mexico, the Zuni tribe makes crystal fetishes that are representative of animal spirits. These fetishes are nourished and fed with a mixture of ground maize and powdered turquoise. While the beautifully carved fetishes are loved and popular today, the religious ceremony of feeding them is not practiced anymore.

- Turquoise is commonly revered as sacred by many other Native American tribes.

- The Aborigines of Australia and the Maoris of New Zealand continue to practice traditions and religious ceremonies using gemstones and crystals for healing and protection. Some of them are private ceremonies while other traditions are shared with outsiders too.

One of the most interesting aspects of the use of crystals for healing and protection is that the significance and meaning of multiple stones are common across different cultures that have little or no connection with each other. For example, jade is not only considered highly sacred by the Chinese but they also believe that this stone has kidney-healing powers. The Mayans and Aztecs who lived in faraway South American civilizations also had the same belief.

Turquoise is a stone worn for its health and strength-giving properties all over the world. Jasper is another stone that is believed by many cultures to have the power to render strength and peace on the wearer.

The New Age of Crystal Healing

Referred to as the New Age, since the 1980s, crystal healing has seen a revival of sorts. A lot of observations made on crystals using energy-channelizing techniques have revealed the subtle but unmistakable healing powers of gemstones. Moreover, books written on crystals by authors like Michael Gienger and Katrina Rafaell have revived interest in the mysterious powers of gemstones.

Today, crystal therapies are very popular, and have crossed religious and spiritual boundaries as an increasing number of people are unabashedly trying out the healing and protective powers of crystals and gemstones. It would be naive not to make an effort to at least learn about the superpowers contained within the aura of crystals formed over millennia by absorbing some of the limitless strength of nature and the universe.

Why and How Do Crystals Work?

Crystals are formed beneath the surface of the earth over many, many years. They are created in mineral-rich corners of the earth's deep insides with molten rock bubbling away continuously. When hot, molten rocks within the earth's depths come in contact with cooler surroundings, they get solidified into crystals. Additionally, hot gases carrying rocks leave the rocks behind in a cooler environment.

A perfect crystal is created when the external factors like the temperature and pressure are in a harmonious relationship with each other. It is believed that there is a mysterious kind of alchemy that takes place beneath the earth during the formation of crystals. Like most things in nature, the aura surrounding their formation and the beauty of the outcome are crucial factors that make crystals behave the way they do.

Multiple research studies have proven that the entire universe and everything in it including crystals is made up of energy vibrations. The energy inherent in a crystal is used for various purposes including for healing. The energy within the crystals works like that of a magnet attracting certain forces and repelling others.

The energy trapped in the formation of crystals is the secret to their working. Traditional healers know how to harness this trapped energy to be used as required by human beings. Certain types of energy are tangible and can be experienced in an obvious manner by all kinds of people. However, some forms of energy are subtle to the point that only those individuals who have keen energy-sensing powers can feel, experience and harness them. The energy within crystals belong to the second type.

Just to give you an analogy, some people can see through a painting and can tell exactly what the painter was trying to say, right? Many others are likely to see the same painting as meaningless and purposeless. So, who is right, here? Both are right in their own ways because each believes that he or she is experiencing. Therefore, unless you are ready to open your heart and mind to the healing power of crystals, it is likely to remain hidden from you.

Science cannot explain all the subtle layers that participate in the healing power of crystals because science is a new domain compared to the eons of time that have passed through the history of mankind. Science is still in its nascent stage, and the entire universe and its powers are yet to be discovered and understood.

Therefore, if you choose to look at the healing powers of crystals only through a scientific viewpoint, you are quite likely to be left without answers for many of your questions. However, if you choose to believe in the power of nature and her ability to do wonders, then you can access the healing power of crystals too.

The structural quality of each crystal determines which part of your body it is most suitable for. For example, the structure of the rose quartz is aligned with the energy structure of the human heart, and therefore, can be used to clear and cleanse the heart chakra of negative energies and other issues. Like this, each chakra has its own set of crystals that enhance or negate its power.

Chapter 6: The Practical Ways To Use Healing Crystals For Physical, Mental, Emotional And Spiritual Healing

Apart from laying the healing crystals on your chakras, there are other practical ways to use them. These methods are so easy that you can conveniently incorporate them in your daily routine.

Use the crystals as part of your daily ensemble.

More than just making a fashion statement, you can harness the crystal's healing power as you wear them throughout the day. Crystals are often made into jewelry or brooches, but if you wish, you may keep them in a small pouch and attach the bag inside your garments. For ages, people have been using crystals as amulets for protection. If you want to receive energy from the universe, then carry the stone on the left side of your body.

That said, in order for this method to be effective, it has to be in direct contact with or near the body part that needs to heal. For example, if you're suffering from a broken heart, wear an emerald as a pendant, but be sure that the chain is long enough so that the crystal touches the center of your chest (heart chakra). By doing so, you are actively guiding the crystal's healing energy.

Sleep with your crystals tucked under your pillow.

This is advisable, especially if you are suffering from insomnia or night terrors. To ward off bad dreams, use hematite, ruby, or smoky quartz. To fight insomnia, place a lepidolite or a selenite under your pillow.

Additionally, keeping crystals underneath your pillow will enable you to feel more revitalized upon waking.

For those who want to remember their dreams, placing a garnet beneath their pillow can help. Meanwhile, those who wish to experience astral travel can use crystals like Amethyst and Brown Jasper.

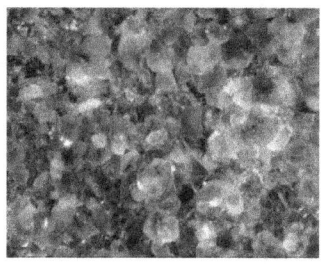

Figure 2 When placed beneath one's pillow, Amethysts are believed to aid in Astral Travel.

Source:

Incorporate crystals in your bath.

Bathing is a form of cleansing not just for the physical body, but also for the other layers of your energy field. Crystals enhance this purging effect by absorbing the negative energies that you've managed to collect throughout the day. To make a warm bath more relaxing, arrange a combination of rose and clear quartz around the tub. Alternatively, you may place the stones in your bathwater. After stepping out of the bath, you'll feel calmer and more revitalized.

Use crystals to boost the power of your meditation.

As previously mentioned, the crystal's stable structure has the power to lend you the balance you need. During meditation, you can achieve stillness and inner peace much easier with the aid of crystals. You may clasp the stones inside your hands or simply set them in front of you.

Concoct gem water or crystal elixirs.

Procedures for making gem water:

Obtain natural spring water and keep it in a glass bowl.

Submerge the crystals overnight.

Keep the gem water in a dark tinted glass bottle with a sprayer and use it as a mist. Alternatively, you may instill a few drops into your bathwater.

Note: Not all crystals are safe to use. There are those that are highly toxic, thus, they are not recommended for use when making gem water. Some crystals should not be absorbed by the skin, let alone be ingested. Some crystal essences, however, are safe enough to be taken in small and diluted amounts.

Procedures for Making Crystal Elixir:

Obtain a bowlful of natural spring water.

Submerge the crystals then place the bowl under direct sunlight. The sunlight activates the memory of the water so that it may absorb the crystal's powerful pattern.

Leave it there for a couple of hours.

Next, get the concentrated essence and keep it in a glass bottle. This is known as the mother essence. Just be sure to fill only half of the bottle.

The other half should be filled with brandy.

Place a few drops of the mixture into a new glass bottle. Afterwards, add drinking water until the bottle is half-filled.

After that, pour brandy into the glass bottle until it's filled.

Drink tiny sips of your crystal elixir throughout the day. If you don't wish to drink it, you may opt to simply inhale the crystal essence.

Decorate your home or your work space with crystals.

Arranging crystals around your home or office will not only brighten and beautify it, but also cleanse it. Crystals can neutralize the negative energies in any environment. More than that, their repeating pattern has the power to inspire harmony. Opt for bigger raw crystals as décor because compared to smaller ones, they are better in maintaining the integrity of their own energy. Thus, they can absorb and trap in negative energies more effectively. As a consequence, they require less cleaning in the future.

Synthetic materials (ex. plastic), electricity, radio waves and microwaves all pose a threat to one's internal and external wellbeing. Manmade substances tend to interfere with natural frequencies. As a result, the earth's natural energy is diminished. We are inevitably exposed to these harmful substances on a daily basis - from our gadgets to our furniture to our simulated lighting. With the use of healing crystals, you can boost your personal energy field, thus, shielding you from the undesirable effects of these energy contaminants.

Procedures for Making a Crystal Grid

Crystals are powerful enough when used alone, but when you make a crystal grid, you can combine their energies and healing powers, thus, strengthening the power of your intention.

To make a crystal grid, you need to determine what your specific intention is. Is it to boost your physical health? To relieve stress? To get rid of depression? To heal a damaged ego? To move on from a painful past relationship? To find spiritual completeness?

This step is important because your intention will help you determine the crystals you will choose for your grid. For instance, intentions of good physical wellness ought to include blue and purple stones such as Sodalite. Intentions concerning matters of the heart may include a combination of malachite and rose quartz. That said, don't discount the power of your instincts when selecting crystals for your grid.

Once you've clarified your intention, the next step is to choose the location of your crystal grid. It would be wise to keep it in a safe area where it's not in danger of being moved. Even so, be sure to keep it where you can see it often.

Next, clear the room's energy. One way to do this is to burn sage. Another would be to put some natural sea salt in a small glass bowl and place it in the center of the room.

Lay a grid cloth on the area. Your intention should be clear enough to be written down in one sentence. Write your intention on a small piece of paper then lay it on the center of the grid cloth.

Breathe in deeply. Vocalize your intention so that your subconscious mind can hear it. Close your eyes and in your mind's eye, see yourself achieving that goal. If your intention is to lose weight then imagine yourself with your new figure. For example, you can envision yourself wearing smaller size clothes and fitting in them, working out and achieving your new body, and stepping on a scale and looking at the numbers in satisfaction.

Arrange the crystals around your intention beginning from the outside moving in.

Each time you add a crystal to your grid, fortify your intention by concentrating on it. With each crystal that you add, feel yourself being one step closer to your goal.

You'll need a center crystal. Lay the final stone down reverently on top of the piece of paper with your intention.

Once you're done, activate your crystal grid. With a quartz crystal, trace the imperceptible line connecting each crystal with the one beside it. Start from the outside moving in.

The last step is to light a few candles around the grid. Once again, think of your intention. Know that your dream is about to come true soon. Feel it with every fiber of your being. Then, snuff out the candles and leave the grid undisturbed for one month and ten days.

Chapter 7: Overview On Crystal Therapy

Crystal therapy or Precious stone treatment is a treatment that is utilized to give fix to different maladies like torment and stress. The quick pace way of life and long working hours have brought forth sicknesses like pressure, uneasiness and body torment. This is an extremely compelling system that helps a ton in giving unwinding. This treatment has been being used since the days of yore.

In the precious stone treatment, the stones and gems are broadly utilized. It is accepted that these gems help in giving the recuperating impacts on the body. A portion of the stones and precious stones are accepted to have the recuperating nature. These stones and gems are put on the viable part so as to give a restoring impact.

There are various sorts of precious stones, each loaded up with their own recuperating capacities for the brain, body, and soul. They're thought to advance the progression of good vitality and help free the body and psyche of negative vitality for physical and passionate advantages.

Truly, gems are touted as old types of medication, with methods of reasoning obtained from Hinduism and Buddhism. In any case, realize that there's no logical proof to help the utilization of gems. Regardless of this, individuals are as yet attracted to their hues and magnificence.

This recuperating treatment is fundamentally a pseudo science. There is no logical verification for this recuperating system. Be that as it may, it is broadly utilized so as to give the unwinding impact. These precious stones when applied on the skin, gives an alleviating impact. The science behind this recuperating treatment is that it animates the skin cells. At that point, this in the long run outcomes in the outflow of the proteins and hormones that help in giving unwinding.

It is accepted that the compelling force of nature has remedy for different infirmities. There are different normally happening substances that contain certain mending properties. These precious stones are utilized so as to have a mending impact. These gems are utilized to give the reviving impact on the body.

The working standard of gem treatment is basic. In this, the stones and gems are given on the territory of the body that is influenced by the torment. These work on the vitality networks of the body. The precious stones are utilized to expel the antagonistic and negative vitality. These inevitably bring about giving restoring impact on the body.

There are different specialists that are offering precious stone treatment. Despite the fact that it has not been demonstrated experimentally to this give has certain mending impact or not. However, the enormous utilization of this treatment superbly mirrors its advantages. This treatment has given medical advantage to a great many individuals. Along these lines, we can't infer that this treatment doesn't have any favorable position.

You can utilize the precious stone treatment to get ideal help from the agony. The stones and gems are put on the various pieces of the body having affected from the agony. This treatment is additionally exceptionally successful in giving unwinding. The gems and stones in the warmed structure are taken care of on the head to give unwinding. The shrouded mending intensity of the stones helps in expelling the pressure and stress. This in the long run outcomes in giving a calming impact on the psyche.

One extremely intriguing reality related with gem treatment is that it doesn't demonstrate any symptom. One takes this treatment so as to dispose of pressure and torment. This is a viable method which can lessen torment without giving any symptom on the body. The normal stones and gems will improve your wellbeing measures.

Gems have been utilized all through all of history as a wellspring of mending power. Old societies everywhere throughout the world utilized recuperating precious stones and stones to adjust, clear and change their vitality, soul and physical wellbeing. The supernatural forces of gems were no secret to most antiquated societies including the Egyptians, Mayans and Sumerians who normally embellished their bodies, gems and structures with these consecrated stones.

Precious stones have been utilized all through all of history as a wellspring of mending power. Antiquated societies everywhere throughout the world utilized recuperating precious stones and stones to adjust, clear and change their vitality, soul and physical wellbeing. The mystical forces of precious stones were no secret to most old societies including the Egyptians, Mayans and Sumerians who normally decorated their bodies, adornments and structures with these holy stones.

How Does Crystal Healing Work?

Investigation into the structure of the particle in the course of the last couple of hundred years has uncovered that everything in our whole universe is comprised of vitality. Indeed, even strong articles, similar to a household item or the hair on your head, are extremely only vibrations of vitality at the most major levels. It may not seem as though it to your eye, yet mending gems and the cells in your body are comprised of a similar sort of vitality.

Researchers have just made sense of how to utilize the vitality intrinsic in precious stones for a wide range of things like keeping time utilizing little quartz gems in your watch or making the electronic segments to your PC and cell phone. Regardless of whether you understand it or not, the fiery properties of mending precious stones and stones are generally utilized in our cutting edge innovation.

We even use gems in our prescriptions. Numerous pharmaceuticals are made by crushing minerals that structure within mending precious stones. Despite the fact that our way of life has a few uses for the fiery properties of precious stones, we have fail to institutionalize their utilization in lively recuperating.

Much the same as magnets use vitality to pull in or repulse, mending stones gems use vitality similarly. At the point when you place certain precious stones over specific pieces of your body, your vitality changes, vibrates, heartbeats, moves and moves as per the properties and vivacious mark of the gem.

What Type of Healing Can You Expect From Crystals?

You can utilize precious stones to mend everything from headaches to nervousness and past. Recuperating precious stones can likewise quicken your reflection rehearses, adjust your 7 crystals and even instigate daze states under the correct conditions. There's no restriction to the sorts or level of recuperating you can get from the correct precious stone or stone in the correct application.

In case you're hoping to recuperate some part of your psyche, body or soul, there are basically 3 essential ways mending gems can change your vitality and resolve lopsidedness:

Clearing — Crystals can assimilate and expel particular kinds of vitality from your body. Like a magnet can get little bits of metal shavings, a mending precious stone can ingest negative vitality from your body.

Stimulating – Healing gems and stones can likewise push vitality into your body, brain or soul through inciting full frequencies. This is like the manner in which power works by directing and moving vitality into an article. A precious stone can saddle vitality from the quantum field and send it into your own vitality field. Try not to stress, in contrast to power, this gem recuperating vitality is easy and not perilous.

Adjusting – Our reality is even. Take a gander at the leaves on trees or even your body. The vitality of our planet adjusts things in a reflected example. Now and then, your vitality might be skewed and out of equalization, and recuperating precious stones can utilize the properties referenced above, which are basically drawing in and repulsing, to adjust zones of enthusiastic disharmony.

Approaches to Use Healing Crystals

There are tons of kinds of mending stones and gems on the planet. There is a mind boggling measure of undiscovered mending power simply sitting out there hanging tight for you! In any case, before we jump into making sense of what kind of precious stone is perfect for your own utilization, how about we go over some various ways you can utilize gems to recuperate yourself.

Wear mending gems. Since gems and stones assimilate, repulse and transmit vitality, wearing certain recuperating gems can enable you to adjust your vitality field for the duration of the day. Think about the precious stones you wear like taking a nutrient. You eat the nutrient and it sustains your body for the whole day. Putting on your precious stone adornments in the first part of the day or placing certain stones in your pocket resembles taking your day by day nutrient on a vigorous level.

Spot recuperating gems on a particular piece of the body. Anybody acquainted with gem recuperating is most likely acquainted with this kind of mending—the laying of stones. In case you're searching for an immediate, explicit application, setting gems on that piece of your body is a phenomenal method to get to their recuperating properties. For instance, when you get a consume, you apply a consume treatment to the injury. On the off chance that you have a migraine, you may sit discreetly with a quartz precious stone on the spot of your agony.

Contemplate with them. Recuperating stones and gems are frequently a large number of years old, and they contain a ton of data about our history. Truth be told, a quartz gem can hold as a lot of information as more than 22,000 iPhones, and that data doesn't debase after some time. By sitting with gems and calming your brain during reflection, you are regularly ready to naturally get stunning, extraordinary bits of knowledge by essentially grasping a vivacious bit of history like that during the procedure.

Utilize a recuperating precious stone matrix. At the point when you utilize a gem lattice, you spread out explicit sorts of precious stones and stones in a foreordained example. These examples are intended to get and transmute vitality. Utilizing a precious stone matrix is an old recuperating procedure and it can require some investment to gain proficiency with all the various kinds of networks, however the vast majority see it as justified, despite all the trouble as it is an amazingly ground-breaking practice.

Rest close to them. Our intuitive personalities assume control over when we're dozing, and it's an incredible time to mend and learn at a quickened pace. Enabling recuperating gems to work while you're resting can kill any obstacles your normal personality may give dread or uncertainty. Have a go at putting precious stones under your pad or on your bedside table and perceive how they influence your fantasies and how you feel when you get up in the first part of the day.

Move them around the body. Precious stones don't have to sit still to work viably. Truth be told, now and again it's smarter to move stones and precious stones all around your body to get the most mending impact from them. Have a go at utilizing a recuperating precious stone wand to clear negative vitality fields from your head to your toe. Remember that your vitality field stretches out around 3 ft. around you, so don't spare a moment to take a shot at your whole air when rehearsing precious stone mending.

Spot them in your home or vehicle. You can likewise utilize mending stones and precious stones to secure you or enable an aim. For instance, you can put defensive precious stones in your vehicle to square negative vitality from mishaps or break ins by setting that aim into the gem and afterward leaving in them in those spots. You can utilize them similarly in your home or to set the vitality for a room. Precious stones like rose quartz can likewise attract sentimental vitality in your room or mending vitality close to your tub.

Purifying and Aligning Your Crystals

Since mending precious stones ingest, pull in and repulse particular kinds of vitality, it's imperative to keep your gems clean. In the event that you use gems to retain negative vitality, you'll need to dispose of that vitality before utilizing them once more. Think about this like utilizing a wipe to absorb grimy water. In the event that you need to continue utilizing the wipe, you'll have to crush out the filthy grimy water and tidy it up so the following plate you wash doesn't likewise get messy.

At the point when you buy mending gems or stones in a store or on the web, they have been engrossing and repulsing the vitality of everybody who has contacted them. Before you use them on yourself, you'll have to rinse their vitality and adjust it to yours.

Doing this is basic. You can douse your precious stones (don't drench selenite or golden however as they will break down) in cleansed water, salt water or blessed water. Smirching (utilizing the smoke from white savvy, dried herbs or incense) can likewise scrub your precious stones. A few people even give their recuperating precious stones a moon shower by giving them a chance to sit out around evening time under the light of the full moon.

After you've cleaned your stones and gems for recuperating, adjust them to your vitality by holding them in the palm of your hand, shutting your eyes, expressing your goal for them and saying thanks to them for the mending they will give.

At long last, clean your precious stones after each utilization. This implies precious stones you wear each day ought to be cleaned before you wear them the following day, and gems utilized for a recuperating session ought to be immediately cleaned after every session.

Choosing Which Type of Crystal To Use

Counseling a precious stone recuperating aide is an extraordinary method to make sense of which gems to use for which issues and situations. We've included one beneath to kick you off. Be that as it may, your instinct will consistently be your best guide. You can ask the gem or stone how they need to be utilized, reflect with it, utilize a pendulum or essentially go with your first impulse.

Simply don't ponder it. Your reasonable personality doesn't generally have the foggiest idea about the appropriate response, however your intuitive personality does. Utilize your instinct and sense and you'll normally settle on the ideal decision.

White/Clear: Clearing

Models: Quartz, Moonstone, Selenite

Utilizations: White and clear recuperating precious stones are permeable. They are ideal for learning and purging any kind of vitality. Numerous individuals utilize clear quartz in their contemplation rehearses in light of the fact that it clears and quiets the psyche. Make certain to clean your quartz as often as possible since they do ingest to such an extent.

Darker: Allowing

Models: Tiger's Eye, Petrified Wood, Halite

Utilizations: Brown recuperating precious stones and stones are very establishing. At the point when you consider darker gems, think about a soil way in obscurity woods. This way demonstrates to you the way and secures you on your voyage. That is the thing that dark colored stones do—control, secure and make room. Use them when you're attempting to make room in your life for something like a new position or relationship.

Red: Energizing

Models: Ruby, Garnet, Jasper

Utilizations: Red mending gems have a great deal of vitality. You can help yourself to remember this by thinking about your response to a red stop sign, a red traffic light or a red admonition sign. Red conjures abrupt floods of vitality, so on the off chance that you need a speedy lift me up, you can bear a red stone as a substitute for something undesirable like a jazzed drink.

Orange: Releasing

Models: Copper, Sunstone, Aragonite

Utilizations: You know when you feel truly wiped out and you venture into the daylight and feel much improved? That is on the grounds that orange is at the same time a relieving and stimulating shading. Orange mending stones discharge negative vitality and get out space for an increase in wellbeing vitality. Use them when you're feeling sad or you're stalling.

Yellow: Aligning

Models: Amber, Sulfur, Mookaite

Utilizations: Yellow gemstones are extraordinary for revamping vitality designs. These recuperating precious stones are ideal for times when you're attempting to impart another propensity or break an unfortunate one. Consider yellow stones like an extremely productive made. They don't simply purge vitality, they rearrange it.

Green: Balancing

Models: Jade, Emerald, Malachite

Utilizations: Green gemstones are frequently utilized for physical recuperating as a result of their adjusting properties. Frequently, our sicknesses involve a lot of something. For instance, stomach related problems frequently come from an excessive amount of corrosive or a lot of undesirable microbes. While we need these things to endure, a lot of them makes us wiped out. Green mending stones don't dispose of negative vitality; rather, they tip the scales the correct way, diverting our vitality streams and adjusting them.

Blue: Communicating

Models: Sapphire, Sodalite, Angelite

Utilizations: Just like the blue throat crystal, blue mending precious stones are about transparency and correspondence. In case you're experiencing difficulty finding your fact, or you need reality to be uncovered about something, work with blue precious stones for recuperating.

Indigo: Calming

Models: Kyanite, Azurite, Lapis Lazuli

Utilizations: Sometimes, as gets extremely riotous and you simply need to unwind and relax. Next time you need to get yourself a quieting spa experience, utilize the relieving intensity of dim blue/indigo recuperating gemstones to relax on edge, delicate vitality.

Violet: Uplifting

Models: Amethyst, Iolite, Sugilite

Utilizations: Violet is one of the most dominant hues, since it vibrates at a high recurrence/wavelength. It is at the highest point of our shading range, consolidating both the warm and cool parts of the bargains hues we can see. Along these lines, anything violet associates you to higher plane of presence. Violet recuperating precious stones are no special case, and they are immaculate it you should be inspired, need to initiate an otherworldly encounter or approach higher forces to direct you.

Dark: Protecting

Models: Tourmaline, Apache Tears, Obsidian

Utilizations: Black recuperating precious stones divert everything. They are solid and versatile, so they make immaculate securing precious stones. On the off chance that you need to repulse any sort of vitality, utilize dark stones to drive those negative energies from you.

Pink: Loving

Models: Rose Quartz, Morganite, Rhodonite

Utilizations: Pink makes us consider sentiment, and that is on the grounds that the shading pink is a blend of energetic red and explaining white. In any case, you don't need to utilize pink mending precious stones only for sentiment. They vibrate a caring, cherishing vitality, so use them for anything that needs a tad of sweetness. They're incredible for redirecting outrage, attracting sentiment or simply making you feel the adoration.

Various kinds of mending gems

Clear quartz

This white precious stone is viewed as an "ace healer." It's said to intensify vitality by retaining, putting away, discharging, and controlling it. It's likewise said to help fixation and memory. Physically, clear precious stones are professed to help animate the insusceptible framework and equalization out your whole body. This stone is frequently matched with others like rose quartz to help and upgrade their capacities.

Rose quartz

Similarly as the shading may propose, this pink stone is about affection. It's said to help reestablish trust and concordance in every unique sort of connections while improving their nearby associations. It's likewise professed to help give solace and quiet during times of anguish.

It isn't about other individuals, however. Rose quartz is said to likewise support love, regard, trust, and worth inside one's self — something we could all utilization nowadays.

Jasper

This smooth precious stone is known as the "incomparable nurturer." It's said to enable the soul and bolster you through occasions of worry by setting you up to completely "appear." It's professed to shield you from and assimilate negative vibes while advancing mental fortitude, brisk reasoning, and certainty. These are qualities that are extra useful when handling significant issues — which is actually what this stone might be useful for.

Obsidian

A strongly defensive stone, obsidian is said to help structure a shield against physical and enthusiastic pessimism. It's likewise said to help dispose of enthusiastic blockage and advance characteristics of solidarity, clearness, and empathy to help locate your actual feeling of self. For your physical body, it might help in absorption and detoxification while possibly decreasing torment and issues.

Citrine

Bring bliss, marvel, and energy to all aspects of your existence with citrine. It's said to help you discharge negative characteristics from your life like dread, and thusly help energize hopefulness, warmth, inspiration, and clearness. It's likewise professed to improve careful characteristics, similar to imagination and focus.

Turquoise

This blue precious stone has powers that are said to help recuperate the brain, body, and soul. As a rule, it's viewed as a four leaf clover that can help balance your feelings while finding your profound groundings. With regards to the body, it's said to profit the respiratory, skeletal, and invulnerable framework.

Tiger's eye

In case you're needing a power or inspiration help, this brilliant stone might be for you. It's said to help free your psyche and assortment of dread, uneasiness, and self-question. This can be valuable for vocation desires or even issues of the heart. Tiger's eye is additionally said to help control you to concordance and equalization to enable you to clarify, cognizant choices.

Amethyst

This purple stone is said to be extraordinarily defensive, mending, and decontaminating. It's guaranteed it can help free the psyche of negative considerations and deliver quietude, earnestness, and profound intelligence. It's likewise said to help advance collectedness. Rest is another asserted advantage of this stone, from as far as anyone knows supporting in a sleeping disorder help to getting dreams.

Physically, it's said to help hormone creation, scrub blood, and assuage agony and stress.

Moonstone

Known for "fresh starts," moonstone is said to support inward development and quality. When beginning new, this stone is indicated to likewise mitigate those uneasy sentiments of stress and insecurity so you're ready to push ahead effectively. It's additionally professed to advance positive reasoning, instinct, and motivation while delivering achievement and favorable luck.

Bloodstone

This incredible mending stone satisfies its name. Bloodstone is professed to help wash down the blood by drawing off terrible natural energies and improving course. Carefully, it supports magnanimity, imagination, and vision while helping you live inside the present minute. It's additionally said it can likewise enable you to free yourself of sentiments of fractiousness, forcefulness, and eagerness.

Sapphire

This blue stone is one of insight and sovereignty. It's said it can draw in thriving, satisfaction, and harmony while opening up the psyche to acknowledge excellence and instinct. Concerning physical wellbeing, this stone is guaranteed to likewise help recuperate eye issues, cell levels, and blood issue while additionally facilitating misery, nervousness, and a sleeping disorder.

Ruby

A red champion, this stone reestablishes essentialness and vitality levels. This can help improve things, for example, arousing quality, sex, and acumen. It's additionally said to help bring mindfulness and the acknowledgment of truth to one's psyche. Rubies were utilized in old occasions to help expel poisons from blood and improve the general circulatory framework.

The most effective method to choose your precious stone

First of all: Identify what you feel you're missing before investigating what stones can give you. This will enable you to demonstrate what's happening inside yourself before relying upon outside sources.

From that point, simply let your instinct pick what's best for you. Regardless of whether a precious stone grabs your attention or you can feel a physical draw toward one, your inward intuitive will help control you to the gem that is directly for you. When it's select, you can make the association you need.

Step by step instructions to think about your precious stone

At the point when you initially bring your precious stone home, you'll need to purify away any pessimism it might have grabbed. You can hold it under chilly, running water from a tap or flush it in a characteristic wellspring of water. In any case, be certain the water is cool, not warm or hot.

Include a touch of ocean salt to the wash down or consume sage to truly enable it to dispose of undesirable energies. You can likewise forget about it to dry in morning daylight or full moon light to let the light channel through.

It's not just about their physical consideration, however. For gems to do something amazing, you rationally need to evacuate the negative vitality or wariness you may have about their capacities. It's essential to regard what they can accomplish for you.

Precious stone extras

The fundamental advantage of precious stones might be their recuperating capacities. However, in case we're by and large totally straightforward, they're likewise extremely wonderful. So it's nothing unexpected individuals make huge amounts of extras out of them, similar to adornments or home designs. Not exclusively will the gems look pleasant, keeping great vitality around never hurt anybody.

Petition dots

Precious stone petition dabs are worn against the heart to rouse a wide range of positive emotions, regardless of whether it be expectation, boldness, or harmony. They're an incredible path for anybody to bear the mending forces of precious stones.

Adornments

Adornments is another incredible method to join a precious stone's capacities. Also, it additionally enables you to flaunt each stone's magnificence.

Napkins

These dazzling napkins are produced using real gemstones from Brazil. The agate stone in this family unit thing will help advance parity and concordance inside the home. These are perfect for the individuals who need to bring great energies into their dwelling place.

Sex toys

These gem sex toys blend their energies with your sexual vitality to help give unadulterated, sexual joy. They're extraordinary instruments for those who've been in a sexual trench to enable them to get open up.

Funnels

In all honesty, you can even clear out of precious stone made hand channels. They're smooth, simple to utilize, and tough. This makes them an incredible present for any individual who uses medicinal weed to deal with a wellbeing condition.

Water bottles

Stylish water containers are similarly as popular as precious stones presently, so it's nothing unexpected the two have been converged into one. In the base of these wonderful glass containers sits a "jewel case." It's said to advance everything from health and magnificence to adjust. This is the ideal accomplice to bring to your next yoga practice.

Takeaway

In the event that you're now incredulous about these mending precious stones, at that point they likely won't benefit you in any way. They're probably not going to do you any damage, however. While there's no logical proof for precious stones, that hasn't prevented individuals from difficult them.

A receptive outlook is critical to acquiring the positive characteristics these wonderful stones can offer. Regardless of whether it's general great vitality you need or explicit recuperating powers, there's nothing amiss with giving precious stones a genuine attempt. Who knows — you may be enjoyably shocked.

Consider Using Crystal Therapy to Survive the Daily Grind

Life can be very upsetting now and again. Getting down to business each and every day and taking care of different duties can for all intents and purposes channel the vitality out of you. You can feel baffled with day by day dissatisfactions that can go from ailment, proficient issues, and love issues and even from the weights of a coming test or an advancement. In the event that you need to take a mending break from these things, at that point you can utilize gem treatment. You can utilize it to get help in recuperating ailment, in adjusting energies, in shielding yourself from negative energies and even in discovering love in this world. Here are some significant focuses that you should think about precious stone treatment.

The Basics of Crystal Therapy

The confidence in precious stone treatment depends on the conviction that specific gems and appeal stones have a ton to do with the adjusting of energies inside us. Obviously, it is likewise determined to the possibility that we as a whole have a sort of vibration vitality framework and the utilization of these appeal stones and precious stones can d a lot to block this framework out. As such, these stunning stones have recuperating or enchanted powers inside them and we as a whole can utilize them without anyone else's input or however the assistance of a precious stone advisor. The proficiency of this sort of treatment would be put together not just with respect to the capacity to draw a gem's forces out yet additionally in the stone's compound organization, its sort, its shading, its nuclear structure and its over physical structure. This additionally implies a specific precious stone can have explicit unique powers that can reply to specific needs. Be that as it may, the possibility that a solitary appeal stone more often than not contains one sort of mending power as well as a few.

On the off chance that you need to utilize precious stone treatment for different recuperating purposes, at that point here is a straightforward guide about specific gems and appeal stones and their comparing qualities.

1. Crystal Balancers

There are sure precious stones which can help you in the adjusting of your vitality. This is a decent spot to begin in the event that you don't have the foggiest idea yet which region of center you would need. To have a general adjusted nature, at that point you can utilize jade, serpentine and fulgurite as your crystal adjusting stones.

2. Love Crystals

In the event that you need to get help in the territory of affection, at that point you can utilize love precious stones. The most prevalent ones are the rose quartz, apatite and the colbaltocalcite. These appeal stones emit warm and delicate energies so they are ideal to either to draw in affection or even to enable you to be progressively humane to everyone around you.

3. Empowering Charm Stones

On the off chance that you are bit low as far as vitality, at that point you can utilize special necklaces, rings or some other adornments piece with opal or topaz stones as a component of your gem treatment. These appeal stones can help you when you are debilitated and exhausted. Simply make certain to fend off them from your bedside so you can have a decent night's rest.

4. Memory Keepers

There are stones which help the memory hold a lot of data thus they are likewise called gem record attendants. A few models incorporate rubies, garnets and carnelians. They can be very valuable when you are getting ready for tests.

5. Defensive and Shielding Crystals

Jewels, yellow jasper and fluorite are the best defensive appeal stones. They work best when worn as a gems trimming or when kept in the tote or pockets. These gems basically work by retaining the negative energies around you so realizing how to wash down them fro time to time is additionally significant.

The utilization of the previously mentioned precious stones are all piece of gem treatment which for the most part expect to adjust the vitality inside you. Gem treatment is likewise known to recuperate and loosen up the body and brain and furthermore to reinforce the body's insusceptible framework.

Advantage OF CYSTAL THERAPY

Precious stone treatment has been utilized for quite a long time to help treat the body comprehensively for different infirmities and the utilization of these delightful minerals goes back to Egyptian occasions when they were said to be utilized to cleanse 'malicious spirits.'

The conviction behind gem treatment is that individual stones, for example, amethyst, rose quartz and jade can speak with the vitality stream of the human body and help to realign the vitality channels that are intruding on the regular progression of the body and help it recuperate itself. Precious stones with explicit stones are said to alleviate explicit illnesses, for example, nervousness, gloom and a sleeping disorder, or increasingly physical afflictions, for example, stomach related issues.

Gem treatment can be as straightforward as wearing valuable stones and minerals as wristbands and pieces of jewelry, setting precious stones in the room where you work and rest or being treated by a gem advisor, who can recognize which stones can work to invigorate the seven crystals, or 'vitality focuses' around the body.

Chapter 8: Using Crystals For Healing

Boost your Mood with Crystals

For hundreds of years, human civilization has been fascinated by the power of crystals. They are commonly used for harnessing their powerful and healing energies. Crystals can be used to bring about a greater sense of happiness, health, and even heal any deep-rooted issues.

Rose Quartz

The calming and soothing energy of this crystal represents harmony and love. It not only increases your heart to be more loving but makes it easier to receive love and the ability to forgive oneself and others. It is important to move on. If you keep holding onto any petty grudges or hurt, you can never truly form lasting relationships. The equation you share with others often influences the way you feel. If all your relationships are rather troubled, then you will be riddled with insecurities and a variety of negative emotions.

Emotional balance is the precursor to good decision-making. Whenever you need to clear your mind of any emotional troubles, then use this crystal. For instance, when you are in a foul mood, the chances of rational and logical decision making dwindle drastically. One poor decision is all it takes to change the course of your life. Unless you understand your emotions and what they mean, you cannot take charge of them. Instead of living a life regulated by your emotions, learn to regulate your emotions.

This crystal can also be used to heal any emotional trauma and replace it with peace and calm. If you want to create a positive and peaceful vibe in your immediate surroundings, then use rose quartz.

Clear Quartz

The master healer or the clear quartz can be used for pretty much anything and everything. The translucent and clear crystal has the energy to heal any issues associated with your physical, emotional, mental, and even spiritual wellbeing. The energy frequencies of clear quartz resonate with the spiritual chakras. It, in turn, enables the divine light to run through your body and form a connection with the higher self. A combination of these factors enables to usher in unconditional love, wisdom, and a higher sense of conscience is clear. If you often feel like any issues from your past are holding you back, then use a clear crystal to let go of the past. Once you let go of the past, it becomes easier to live in the moment, and it will automatically improve your overall as well. Whenever you are experiencing any extreme mood swings, sit quietly for a while and meditate with clear quartz.

Citrine

Citrine is certainly quite popular, and its yellow-gold color makes it attractive too. Citrine is not just used for its beauty, but the healing properties it possesses. If you want to attract abundance and prosperity into your life, then use this crystal. It is commonly known as the Merchant's stone since it's energy vibrations can help remove any financial obstacles while attracting more opportunities into your life. Financial woes are amongst the leading causes of stress and anxiety. When in a crunch, rational thinking often takes a backseat.

Citrine is commonly used for its protective and creative energy. Place this crystal in a cash drawer or carry it with you to magnify its positive vibrations.

Amethyst

Amethyst is popularly known as the all-purpose stone. It often comes in various shades of violet, ranging from lavender to a vibrant purple. This stone not only resonates with the Crown chakra but the third eye chakra as well. If you're looking for a gateway to higher levels of integration and an understanding of the divine consciousness, then use this stone.

Amethyst is believed to lend a sense of clarity whenever there is chaos in mind. At times, all it takes is a little clarity to let go of anxiety or stress. If you are dealing with extreme mood swings, problems with the immune system, and insomnia, then Amethyst can be quite helpful. Amethyst is also known as the Traveler's Stone and provides protection, while the wearer is on the road or exploring any new places.

Black Tourmaline

This crystal is often used for protecting one's aura. It's also amongst the best protective stones available. The energy it generates will make you feel grounded while creating an energy shield around you to protect from the adverse effects of electromagnetic fields. The best way to use this stone is to place it around electronic devices or gadgets to protect yourself from the EMF frequencies. You can place it at your home and workplace to reduce the presence of any negative vibrations in your immediate surroundings. Not just that, but if there is any negative energy directed towards you and harmful intentions, then this stone can protect you. Any negativity present around you can be immediately transformed into positivity by using this stone. Associated with your goals or dreams, then this crystal can bring about a sense of positive energy and abundance with that.

Aventurine

It is believed to be a lucky stone that comes in different shades of green, peach, blue, yellow, red, and more. It helps attract lasting relationships, love, and friendship into your life. If you're looking for a little added luck in your life, then start using stone. Apart from it, it's also believed that this crystal helps to increase your self-esteem and confidence. While optimizing your chances for growth in life. Since this crystal is often associated with the heart chakra, any emotional issues of the heart can also be healed. The physical effects of this stone can help deal with any sleep disorders, regulate blood pressure, and even any allergies.

Carnelian

This stone comes in a variety of colors ranging from reddish-brown to a very light hue of orange. To feel motivated, confident, and inspired, keep this stone around you. Whenever you feel like you're stuck in a tough spot, this stone will give you the strength and motivation to keep going. Apart from that, it also acts as a natural energy booster why spreading feelings of joy while removing any impure energies present with or around you.

There are several hundreds of crystals with plenty of healing properties, and they come in different colors, sizes, and shapes. Choose a crystal depending upon which of these crystals resonate the most with your beliefs and your needs.

Manifest Health and Happiness

Since centuries various ancient civilizations across the globe have constantly used crystals for removing any mental, spiritual, and physical blockages of energy. Since crystals are obtained from the earth, when placed on the human body, they enable you to connect with the healing energy out by the planet. It tends to make you feel more balanced and relaxed. Every crystal has different properties, and energy is it can be used for healing specific aspects of your life.

Bloodstone for Energy

Bloodstone has been used as an amulet for purifying the plant since ancient times. Whenever the blood and energy present within us are flowing smoothly, we tend to stay healthy and strong. It is an incredible energizer and helps overcome negative thoughts, lethargy, and self-doubt. Apart from that, the bloodstone also stimulates enthusiasm while increasing your drive to be successful in life and helps maintain emotional balance.

Turquoise for Healing

Turquoise is believed to have tremendous healing properties, and if the energetic connection between earth and the cosmos. Since time immemorial, it is amongst the most popular stones used for its protective properties. It is also used as a good luck charm. Whenever a turquoise is given as a gift, the healing properties present within it are magnified. If you have any issues communicating, then wearing turquoise, will improve these issues. It enables you to speak the truth.

Rose Quartz for Love

Rose quartz is commonly associated with the heart chakra. It symbolizes unconditional love and helps stimulate the flow of energy from the heart. It also helps heal any issues associated with love and acceptance. Rose quartz helps cultivate feelings of forgiveness as well. It is quite easy to make mistakes, but forgiving oneself and others for the mistakes made takes incredible strength and courage. It is easy to be critical of yourself and indulges in self-doubt. If you are struggling with self-love or maintaining happy and healthy relationships in your life, then this crystal will come in handy. The energy it emanates helps trigger feelings of unconditional love, care, and nourishment. Rose quartz is the conduit of the most powerful energy present in the universe- love.

Smoky Quartz for Letting Go

Smoky quartz effectively transforms all negative energy into positive ones and is used as a protective shield against negative energy. The key to success is growth, and you cannot grow in life unless you are willing to let go of certain old patterns. If your beliefs are holding you back, then a smoky quartz crystal will come in handy. It helps remove any energy blockages, eliminates stale energy, and revitalizes your body with positive energy. Once all the old energy is successfully eliminated, it creates space for new energy.

Quartz for Clearing Your Mind

Quartz is perhaps the most easily available crystal, and it is abundant in nature. Quartz is essentially made of silica. Silica is an element present in the cells within the human body. Whenever this crystal comes in contact with your skin, it helps merge the energies present within the external world. Therefore, it is believed to promote healing and health. Quartz was commonly used by ancient civilizations to clear the mind while restoring balance to the physical body. It not only successfully amplifies positive energy but removes negative energy. So, it helps raise the vibrations of your personal energy field and lends a sense of clarity to its wearer.

Carnelian for Creativity

Several ancient civilizations strongly believed that carnelians attract good fortune while manifesting one's true desires. It helps remove any blockages in creative energy. Any such blockages can make you feel uninspired and easily drained out. If you are tired of feeling like you are stuck in a rut, then this crystal is the best option available. The vibrant orange color of this crystal is the true representation of the positive and motivational energy it gives out. It helps stimulate your internal reserves of passion and creativity you require to attain your goals. Carnelian brings about feelings of utter joy, confidence, and tremendous motivation.

Celestite For Relieving Stress

Celestite is derived from the Latin word "Caelestis," which translates to celestial. It is believed that even by merely gazing at the pleasant blue hue of this crystal can help trigger happiness and bring about a sense of serenity. If you wish to increase the flow of balancing energy and promote a sense of tranquility, then use this crystal. The best area to place this crystal is in the bedroom. When you place it directly on your body, it acts as a stress reliever. If you notice any stress in a specific region in your body, then use this crystal.

Aventurine for Opportunities

Unless you overcome self-doubt, you cannot see any opportunities life provides you even if it is staring you in the face. By opening up your heart's energy, aventurine helps attract new opportunities into your life. If you struggle with any issues associated with self-worth or cannot let go of your pessimism, then aventurine will come in handy. Once your mind is clear and your energy field is open to receiving energy, you can see opportunities that you never could!

Citrine to Live in the Present

Citrine brings about happiness and light. It has no negative energy present and has tons of positive vibrations. If you struggle to live in the present because you often think about the past or worry about the future, then use citrine. True happiness cannot be attained unless you have self-awareness. Living in the moment and enjoying life is the key to happiness. Apart from this, it also gives you the courage to dream big and keep a positive attitude as you go through life. Once you start giving out positive energy into the universe, the universe will reward you with more positive energy.

Shungite for Protection from EMF

Shungite has been around for millions of years and is abundant in Russia. There is ongoing research to fully understand the true potential and possibilities offered by this crystal. At present, shungite is used as an energy shield against the harmful radiation of the electrical, magnetic energy, or EMF. Shungite helps absorb all sorts of low vibrational energies along with any pollutants. If you work for prolonged periods on any electronic gadgets, then place a shungite next to it. You can also wear it to protect yourself from harmful EMF.

Chapter 9: How Can I Improve My Life With Crystals?

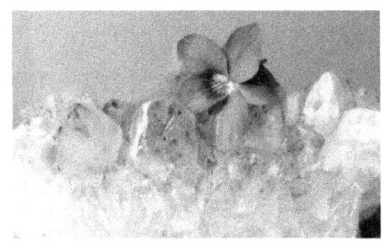

If you have crystals with you and you can sense subtle energies of your crystals, then it is a nice sign that you are improving your life with it. This is a perfect way to create a long-lasting relationship with your stones. This power can help you to feel the universe around you while making you understand its true meaning. If you are getting a hard time to sense the energies of your crystals, then it is a perfect time for you to sense the energy frequency of your body first, to work with it before you jump to crystals. To do that, rub your hands will be the first technique to feel the energy accumulating under it. The next step would be to slowly move your hands apart. After you are done with this, the third part comes when you try to feel the energy of the crystals. Rub your hands and then put any crystal near you. Feel the difference between both your body's energy field and of the crystal.

If you are drawn to purchasing yourself a new crystal, that means that you are curious about stones and you already have one. If you don't, that's not a problem. But if you have crystals already and you want more then it is a good sign that you are improving your life with it and you want to try different stones. Other ways to improve your life with crystals would be to cleanse your stones. The perfect way to cleanse your stones is through the power of your inner guidance. If you are having a hard day emotionally, psychologically, and physically, then you should initiate the process of crystals right away.

If you are in love with your crystals, always using it when it is needed like a habit, then it is a strong sign that you are improving your life with it. This act of dedication allows the spirit to become awakened. If you are doing this, then you are awakening the crystal too with positivity and purpose to provide you back the same, enhancing the intuitive world inside you as well.

Crystals as an antidote

The use of crystals as a medicine has been used for thousands of years. You have to select the crystals to your purpose. It should be aligned with your intention and purpose. Scientifically, there is no proof that stones have the abilities to cure diseases, but many people want to try an alternate method, want to try something new. From allowing positive healing to alleviating any disease-causing energies, it provides you with the choice of what kind of energy that you want to cultivate, including things such as love, intuition, prosperity, fortune, and spiritual awakening, etc.

Having the right crystals with you can give you the needed support, comfort, and can empower you to a major life transformation. Many crystals in their water-infused base provide the solution to different parts of the body, also, including the different chakras. All these things have been discussed above thoroughly. There have been studies done where it proves that the people receiving the treatment of different crystals can have a placebo effect on their system. Just like a patient think that going to the doctor will cure them, the crystal lures think that using stones as medicine will cure them. The belief is so strong that sometimes the placebo effect works very well.

Crystals as an aid for healing the chakras – crystals for anger, stress, and trust.

Chakras are the centre points in the human body. They are swirling wheel carrying light energy, each ranging differently, and which had been discussed above. Sending and receiving universal energies, these charkas are the connection points through which we interact with our world. There are seven chakras point, but there are many minor chakras that are countless and relates to the well-being of mind, body, and soul. If all the chakras are healthy and they are moving with the right flow, then they bring the wellness to the overall human body, but the influence of the external energies sometimes disturb the energy flow of the chakras. Below are the crystals that aids to help with anger, stress, and trust, and which chakras point to place those crystals:

•**Howlite**: Place this over your crown chakra to prepare yourself to receive wisdom and energies to deal with your anger. It allows you to understand the need of nurturing oneself while assisting you to deal with your past anger. Howlite also helps in reducing the anxiety, stress, and tension as well as enhancing the awareness of your mind. It also allows you the way to express your emotions so that the negative energy goes out through venting.

•**Amethyst**: Already being discussed in the mantras section, Amethyst need more elaboration because it is one of the most important crystals out there for healing. Providing spiritual clarification if placed over the third eye, it also relieves the geopathic stress. Providing aid in sadness, it also balances the hormones to get rid of the mood swings, also, helping in addictions. According to Archbishop, this crystal instils the good soul with the thinking of heaven.

•**Black Jasper**: It is best known for lower chakras, this stone provides the necessary physical stability for the person suffering from emotional crisis. Alleviating the pain such as hip-joint, re-balancing the human body's intake, Jasper comes in the wide variety of colours and the different colours provide different uses. Aligning the chakras, it also promotes higher vibration to the body.

•**Himalayan Salt Rock**: Though used in kitchens for a variety of benefits, this crystal connects all the three main chakras such as root, solar plexus, and sacral chakras. Eating and working with this salt provides you to stabilize these chakras. You are practising peace with this crystal. It also helps in easing stress and anger.

•**Pink Smithsonite**: A zinc carbonate crystal, this stone helps in regulating your physical weight, so that it can cope up with your physical energies. It also balances the reproductive system, helping you to build trust in yourself. It also clears out all the chakras.

•**Carnelian**: It provides stimulation to the sacral chakra, giving you the right flow of energy. It heals the kidneys too. With this stone, you can transform the world. It provides you with a natural trust within you to pursue your path as it builds action and courage.

Why should you consider crystal therapy?

Crystal therapy is becoming popular these days because so many books are being published in this subject. People are sharing their experience of using crystals worldwide, so the word is spreading. There are also classes and seminars being conducted to educate the people about the crystal. Crystals are present for millions of years. From Greek mythologies to Archbishop, from Mesopotamians to early Europe, people have a history of using crystals. So, there is something about it that is to be unravelled here. Whether is it your curiosity, or whether you are invested in this 'pseudoscience', you have to find it, you have to experience the enigma of crystals. To investigate crystals might look far-fetched, but the world of science has not dug up into the science behind vibrational frequency and the effects of the vibrational frequency of humans, so it is the responsibility of the individual to explore the world and find his/her ways. Decide it for yourself. Take crystal therapy.

The first thing you can expect in your crystal therapy would be consultation. The person will ask you about the story of you reaching them, everything related to you and your relationship with the crystals. Again, if you are just curious to know about crystals even if you don't have any experience with them, that's fine. Your therapist will ask you all types of questions because the crystal is a holistic subject: it looks at every aspect of the being: every chakra. Once your consultation is over, the therapist will be aware of how to work with you. He or she will use the crystals that will be best for you. He/ she will provide you with all the comfort, while you lie down in a comfortable place. In a relaxed position, the therapist will place the crystals around your body. At this time, you are asked to breathe deeply so that you can relax. Some people feel a tingle here, some don't. You may need to attend more sessions for the overall wellbeing. Just check that your therapist is qualified or not because it is certainly important. Just feel your first experience and decide whether you need more crystal therapy or not. If you have read this far, do go for crystal therapy.

Which physical or psychical diseases crystals help to heal?

There are so many crystals that heal physical and psychical diseases that we have to put them under a sub-category:

- Crystals for anxiety

- **Kunzite**: It is a variety of spodumene. It is pink and semi-rare. Showing striations over the surface of lavender-pink to transparent crystal, it is a monoclinic crystal. Artificially, the mineral in Kunzite amplifies the intensity of its colour. This stone gets its name as Kunzite because it was in honour of the American mineralogist whose name was George Frederick Kunz. This was done in 1903. Carrying no historical significance, in today's world, this crystal promotes bliss and absolute positivity inside the mind. It pushes the negative energy out of your body while promoting a strong heart chakra so that one can manifest contentment and peace in all the aspects of life. This crystal is very sensitive and gentle. It helps in clearing out the anxiety while calming the body down.

This stone realigns your belief in god, universe, and spirits to heal your vibration and to cool down your anxiety, allowing you to be playful. Kunzite tells you to take your responsibilities only when it seems beneficial to you so that you can promote your mental health and overall well-being. Keep this crystal with yourself, especially, during the major things in your life such as promotion, divorce, retirement, career change, etc. Kunzite helps you to see the things with a positive outlook and strengthens the heart chakra.

●**Rose Quartz**: This crystal can transform your relationship with yourself. Brining love and harmony, it heals emotions. If you hold this crystal to your heart, it brings loving vibes to it while providing a higher level of protection. It opens the third eye, giving you the power of strength as well as a deep level of guidance on how to live life, eradicating anxiety. Rose quartz helps to release emotions that are not expressed properly. It also helps to alleviate the psychosomatic diseases. Harmonizing the brain, it also assists in helping in dementia by realigning the neurotransmitters, and also, opening the new neural pathways. If you are unable to recognize your damaged emotions, place Rose Quartz closer to you. Draw closer to feel positive.

●Crystals for abundance

- **Amazonite:** This crystal protects the body from radiation. It pures the individual's electromagnetic field. The vibrations that it distorts also includes the wi-fi. It is said that wi-fi depletes the immune systems of sensitive people. This crystal aligns the nervous system into the calm mod to relieve muscle spasms. It resonates with calcium, which allows the individual to regulate with the calcium intake in the body and balance any deficiencies relating to metabolism. The colour of the Amazonite crystal comes from the lead that explains why it protects the individual from radiation relating to destructive emotional patterns, while also encouraging creative thinking. It allows the person to dive into reality, to live consciously.

- **Clear Quartz**: This crystal works with all the chakras. This is also a neutral crystal. But not only that, it also acts as an amplifier of the vibrational frequency. It clears out the negativity while increasing the spiritual receptiveness. This is an important crystal for abundance because it magnifies the frequencies of the other crystals too. Clear Quartz is very durable and is the crystal to maintain positive energy. It activates the crown chakra, helping in establishing a flow of clarity.

- Crystals for relieving fear

- **Rhodochrosite**: Having different appearances, this crystal has a soft trigonal mineral in it. Having its colours ranging from magenta to red, and from opaque to swirling layers of pink, and from white to the transparent and translucent, this crystal is used for clearing the negativity and karmic wounds from your ancestral lines. The Incas have the notion that this stone has the blood of Incan royalty. This crystal was used to form Incan jewellery for funerary. This crystal is known as Rosinca for this reason. Once every two hundred years, it is said that there is a heart-shaped Rhodochrosite crystal that lay deep below the beats of the Andes that is very sacred. A national crystal for Argentina and a mineral state of Colorado, this crystal removes the pattern of your trauma and karma. Rhodochrosite helps your being, while also taking care of your DNA level. Use this crystal to promote forgiveness in your life and show empathy, so that you can take care of your emotional abuse from this lifetime, or the lifetime relating to your past. From illness and injury, Rhodochrosite restores the cells of your body, while amplifying the energy that surrounds you. It also contains manganese, providing the body with the right metabolic function and giving powerful antioxidant. Manganese can prove toxic if taken in large quantities. Asserting the heart, it eases with the lungs. Placing this at the crown, at the base of the skull, Rhodochrosite might help in opening the blood vessels. Carrying a high vibrational field, this might open the heart chakra for unconditional love. If placed on the crown chakra, this crystal helps you to realize the purpose of your present life existence. It lets you understand the divine within yourself.

•**Malachite**: This crystal came from the copper mines of Egypt that was operated by the Goddess Hathor six thousand years ago. This crystal was used as an amulet to drift the evil eyes and was used for enchantment. Historically, people carved the image of the sun of the stone because they thought this won't allow the black magic to work. In the Pliny, this stone depicts the story that it protected children and nursing mothers. It is the perfect stone for soaking the environmental pollution and transferring energies from one body to another. It helps with radiation, geopathic stress, and the distortion in the electromagnetic field. The Egyptian used this crystal to their eyes by creating its paste, and also, used this for infected wounds. In recent times, Malachite has been found to have an antibacterial property because of the presence of the copper carbonate hydroxide, also, healing arthritis when in the bloodstream. Crystal lures today use Malachite to ease with the individual having psychosexual difficulties. Best used under the experienced guidance, Malachite can also be helpful in meditation or can be placed in the third eye to bring that intense inner transformation. Keep in mind that this crystal is powerful and allows the person to feel its imperfection that one might not like. You have to take responsibility for feelings, thoughts, and actions. This is good for spiritual evolution, making it a marvellous soul and karmic cleanser. Activating your soul's purpose, it gets rid of the trauma and draws spiritual energy that amplifies the vibrational frequency of your soul. Wash your hands properly after using this stone.

Crystal for creativity

•**Tiger's eye**: Roman soldiers used to wear this crystal as armour to deflect the weapons during the war. Wolf stone is the other name for Tiger's eye. This crystal is dedicated to the Mesopotamian God whose name is Belus. This stone defends against curses and regarded as a stone for good fortune provider. The bands of the crystal are built by needles of amphibole that has grown under the quartz. This produces a sharp reflection of light when seen from another direction, and appears black from another direction. This occurs when the crystal is polished. Tiger's eye helps to deflect the negative energy.

This crystal enhances the eye's vision and its overall well-being. It allows you to be agile like the cat's eyes. Yin and Yang's energies get restored while promoting harmony. This had been said in Chinese medicine. It increases the experience of kundalini if placed over the lower chakras. As it holds within it the energy of the sun, it may help to cure depression. It also helps in digestion, to help in lower blood pressure, and increases the healing of broken bones if any. On the head, if the stone is placed on either side of it then it helps to balance the brain. If you are pompous, wearing Tiger's eye will help you to develop personal will as well as helping you with your creativity. If in your life things are not going well according to you, but the environment is not that harsh then this crystal can help you to set realistic goals. Helping your needs and wants with others, this crystal helps you to be not emotional, but logical. If you are uncommitted in your life, then this crystal can assert you in difficult situations. This is the crystal of protection that also evokes your inner vision. You can place this crystal on your reproductive organs to help you with fertility.

•**Orange Kyanite**: This stone looks like crystallized sunshine and was found in Tanzania. Increasing the potential of your creative power, it also helps you with your manifesting abilities. This colour of Orange Kyanite comes from manganese; its scales, when reflecting, that are of golden colour are mica which provides high vibrational frequency as they are an optimal transmitter of energy. The orange colour helps you to dive deep into your psyche and gets off the blockages related to creativity. It activates the sacral chakra by energizing it. It also helps the being to accept that he/she is a sexual being and helps in procreation. This crystal helps to find the right alignment between passion and pleasure.

If the first chakra is blocked, then it results in low self-esteem and inferiority complex creating problems like jealousy or condescending behaviour. If you have with yourself an Orange Kyanite, this crystal can detach these awful things and can start the process of healing. Orange Kyanite can open all chakras, cleansing them, and shining some light on them. This stone can also open psychic channels so that it can manifest spiritual energy while facilitating a higher vibrational frequency. It also helps to alleviate karmic problems from past life, especially, relating to sexual experiences. Orange Kyanite or Kyanite is also known as disthene, a Sanskrit word, meaning 'twice'. The reason it is called twice because it possesses negative and positive polarities.

You should place Orange kyanite to your belly to get rid of any underlying disease such as diabetes, infertility, muscle cramp, allergies, chronic pain, intestinal dysfunction, urinary infection, and chronic back pain. This crystal also helps in unravelling the hidden causes of any addiction, or if somebody has an eating disorder. Orange Kyanite helps the body to realign with its normal functioning. When you have this crystal with you and you are placing this crystal on the sacral chakra for five minutes a day, then you are creating a new world for you. You will have a higher level of creativity, while you take pleasure in love and life. You will become confident and more assertive.

- Crystals for fertility

- **Blue moonstone**: These crystals are found in parts of India and Sri Lanka. The power of Moonstone lies in the connection with the moon. The glossy shine that it has on the surface, it is created by the water in the stone. These stones help in menstruation and menopause. This crystal helps the women to have high positive energy vibration before any conception. It calms the soul. There are White Moonstones too which causes the individuals to have different delusions, but with the help of the Blue Moonstones, these delusions become the gateway for awakening the spiritual potential and expanding the consciousness. There are three types of Moonstones; Blue, White, and Rainbow. All three have different purposes but are used together for balancing the polarities that femininity and masculinity has.

- **Aquamarine**: In Greek mythology, Aquamarine was the powerful seductress who deviated the attention of the sailors from the rock so that they could meet with her. But the man also wore amulets so that they could be safe against the sea monsters and could ensure a safer voyage. The colour of this crystal comes from iron. Aquamarine calms your mind while allowing you to have spiritual awareness. Historically, Christians had a belief that this stone cleansed their sins. Bringing peace of mind, this stone also soothes the women in pregnancy from unnecessary worries and anxieties. Aquamarine allows them to enjoy their beautiful pregnancy confidently, dissolving any questions of self-doubt.

Also good for healing the throat and the vision, this crystal also acts as an antidote against the poison. Balancing the psychic overactivity, it gives clarity to the mental perception. Aquamarine also discourages women to have any thoughts about miscarriage. Place this crystal over your heart to eliminate this fear. Place this crystal over your throat so that you can express yourself better. Promoting tolerance, this is one of the best crystals to have around during pregnancy.

- Crystals to help the reproductive system

- **Aventurine**: It is a healing stone and is versatile. Resonating energetically with the immune system and the thymus gland, this stone also regulates blood; hence, acting as an anti-inflammatory. Green Aventurine works brilliantly with the nervous system, adrenals, heart, and eyes. Blue Aventurine helps in mental healing while enhancing the inner calm. And Peach Aventurine provides the energy flow of the earth into the material body. And Red Aventurine helps in the urogenital system to assist infertility, while also enhancing libido. And White Aventurine helps the neurotransmitters inside the physical body. Aventurine protects the electromagnetic smog to enter inside the body. While also encouraging pregnancy and the improvement of fertility, it helps women with optimism. It pures your heart. This stone also eliminates environmental pollution as well as providing fulfilling abundance. With this stone, you become your true self.

•**Smokey Quartz**: This stone helps to increase the flow of fertility, balancing the sexual energy, while also alleviating the level of depression in both women and men. Stimulating the reproductive organs, this is also an excellent stone for perimenopause and menopause. Also, neutralizing the negative energy vibrations, it eases the digestive system, while helping in alleviating the fear of any kind. This crystal brings back the emotional calmness and reduces the level of anxiety that one experiences. It is one of the most precious and powerful crystals out there, activating the mode of survival instincts. A perfect crystal for cleansing, Smokey Quartz also emits a high vibrational field.

Chapter 10: Individual Gemstones & Crystals

Red, Orange and Yellow Crystals

In this Chapter, we will explore the crystals based on their colors. As you are aware, reds relate to the earth and are grounding, oranges relate to emotions, sexuality, and creativity (and water) and can help heal emotions; and yellows correspond to the solar plexus and bring confidence, self-empowerment, vitality, and will.

We will also be looking at brown and black gemstones in this section due to their connection to the earth element and grounding energies. Once you have developed and integrated an organic understanding of the crystals and their associated properties, this guide should allow you easy and quick access when wishing to jolt your memory (think in terms of color!). Each crystal gemstone has a short description of how it can be used to heal, 'the crystal personality' (the energy of the type of person associated with and strongly resonant to the crystal), key qualities, and the related chakras. I hope this guide will bring you the clarity, wisdom, direction, and healing you desire.

Obsidian

Obsidian is a predominantly black crystal with white or gray markings found in volcanic regions. It is formed from rapidly cooled lava. Due to this birth from the fires within the heart of earth, obsidian is known for its ability to bring, strength, courage, and a sense of practicality and determination.

In addition to its grounding energy, obsidian also has spiritual qualities. It can help release fears and bring hidden emotions to the surface. Deeply buried wounds and traumas can be transformed with obsidian and powerfully brought to light for healing.

Crystal Personality: Emotionally withdrawn or volatile, secretive with an ability to uncover hidden truths and information.

Qualities: Grounding, purging, and transmuting.

Chakra: root

Hematite

Hematite is a very powerful gemstone which connects you to the earth. It is viewed by many as the sacred blood of the Great Mother herself (planet earth). Hematite strengthens the physical body, has a profound effect on the circulatory system and strengthening the blood and can help stabilize systems of the body.

Hematite can help with any feelings of being spaced out or away with the fairies. It brings strength, stability, and grounding and can be connected to balance mind, body, and spirit.

Crystal Personality: Down-to-earth, solid, and dependable. Highly practical with great physical inner strength, however, you may be closed off to subtle, psychic, and spiritual energy.

Qualities: Grounding, stabilizing, strengthening, and practical.

Chakra: root

Black Tourmaline

Black tourmaline is a black, opaque, or slightly translucent gemstone with the ability to bring strength, stability, and grounding. It can be connected to help realign bones and muscles and can aid in adjusting to change in physical life. Tourmaline is formed within the earth's crust, usually deep in fractures.

Black tourmaline can protect you from negative or harmful energy, ill intentions, or destructive vibrations. It can help heal and cleanse your aura through its powerful protective and harmful energy deflecting abilities.

Crystal Personality: Down-to-earth, practical, and connected to your body and the earth. A sense of home being everywhere.

Qualities: Protective, grounding, balancing, and structuring.

Chakra: root

Smoky Quartz

Smoky quartz is a clear yellow-brown crystal, but because of its connection to the root chakra, it is included here. Smoky quartz is found in mountain areas all around the world, usually in crystal filled cavities in rocks. This crystal brings the energy of new beginnings and potential for creativity. It has a grounding, focusing, and gentle healing energy which can be used to both ground and bring security and protection, and energize to spark seeds of change.

Smoky quartz can bring calmness to an overactive mind, release fears and negative thoughts, and aid in meditation. It can teach us to see light in the darkness and brings a deep wisdom through acceptance of our shadow.

Crystal Personality: Strong and quiet energy with deep and creative inner passions. People who resonate with this crystal may lead a quiet and introspective yet highly artistic life.

Qualities: Protecting, grounding, calming, and transforming. Brings change, potential, and new beginnings.

Chakra: root

Red Jasper

Red jasper brings practicality and the energy of the earth. This crystal is formed in the veins and structures of quartz rocks and can be connected to increase focus and bring solid and dependable energy. It is a highly grounding stone yet can also stimulate dreams, psychic abilities, and vision.

Red Jasper can be used for protection.

Crystal Personality: Straightforward and down-to-earth with a grounded and practical energy.

Qualities: Grounding, energizing and stabilizing.

Chakra: root

Bloodstone

Bloodstone is a green gemstone with elements of red. The red spots have been believed through the ages to represent blood hence its powerful connection to the root chakra. Bloodstone is a strengthening stone and can be used to strengthen and stimulate the physical body, circulatory system, and the heart. It can also stimulate a balance of practicality and grounding energy with a desire to grow and expand.

Bloodstone can be used to calm strong emotions and activate life force energy.

Crystal Personality: Courageous and strong individual with intense emotions. You are able to balance your passions with calmness and understanding.

Qualities: Supporting, balancing, circulating, motivating, and calming.

Chakras: root and heart

Garnet

Garnet is usually red, brown, orange, and/or green. It can be connected to spark yourself into inspired action and it brings a very active and fiery energy. Garnet energizes physical processes of the body and can amplify the healing powers of other crystals whilst simultaneously increasing life force.

Garnet can be used to balance any watery or inactive states which need some spark.

Crystal Personality: Busy, obsessive, and impatient. You will often stir things up, sometimes positively, sometimes negatively, however, never subtle.

Qualities: Energizing, activating, and stimulating.

Chakra: root

Carnelian

Carnelian is an orangey-red crystal that brings a gentle yet powerful healing energy. It can be connected with to soothe emotions, release imbalances, and calm stresses and trauma in the sacral chakra. It brings feelings of warmth and connection and can be used to enhance creativity.

Carnelian is gently activating and healing and stimulates the natural healing abilities of the body. It is especially effective for releasing wounds, traumas, and stored emotional pains buried deep within. It can also increase happiness and optimism.

Crystal personality: Friendly, warm, sympathetic and caring personality with emotional wisdom and maturity. You are highly creative, sensual, and sensitive to subtle energy.

Qualities: Soothing, healing, restoring, and transmuting. Brings great creative expression.

Chakra: sacral

Interesting fact: Certain extracts from 'The Book of the Dead' were carved from carnelian and ancient Egyptians recognized the creative and healing energy of this special gemstone. Also, in Greece and Rome, Carnelian was a popular choice for making magical amulets!

Moonstone

Moonstone is a pearl white or blue-white gem for the sacral chakra. It is one of the most powerful stones around to heal and cleanse emotions. It is calming and brings great levels of intuition due to its feminine energy and qualities. Moonstone can quickly release tensions and bring stability to any intense or overactive emotions. On a physical level, moonstone can aid in digestion and digestive upsets and balance fluids in the body.

Moonstone can also increase and develop creativity, empathy, and high levels of intuition.

Crystal Personality: Highly intuitive with a strong connection to one's feminine nature. You may take on a motherly or nurturing role or express oneself creatively.

Qualities: Emotionally balancing, calming, and centering. Develops intuition and natural cycles.

Chakra: sacral

Pearl

Pearl is a gemstone which enhances feelings of tolerance, flexibility, and acceptance. Due to its link to the sea and water, it is very effective for balancing and gently healing emotions. Pearl can stabilize, bring feelings of relaxation, and regulate all bodily functions involving water.

Pearl can ease digestion and release tension and frustration.

Crystal personality: Lover of beauty and depth. Strong emotions, which if expressed positively, can bring great emotional maturity and wisdom.

Qualities: Calming, harmonizing, emotionally energizing, and accepting.

Chakra: Sacral

Tiger's Eye

Tiger's eye is a yellow and golden-brown gemstone formed in between different minerals. It is very powerful for bringing confidence, practicality, and grounding and can be connected to achieve success. It can serve as a great manifestation crystal.

Tiger's eye can also be used to balance the lower chakras and aids in feeling connected to the world. Due to its colors and energetic association with tigers, this crystal can also stimulate joy, lightness of spirit, and feelings of beauty and love for the natural world.

Crystal Personality: Sociable, warm, sunny, and practical with a good sense of humor. You feel comfortable and content in your body and the world around.

Qualities: Grounding, energizing, inspiring, and confidence-building. Sociable, down-to-earth, and practical.

Chakras: root, sacral, and solar plexus. Predominantly solar plexus.

Citrine

Citrine is a transparent yellow crystal with elements of golden brown or orange-brown. It can be used to bring feelings of warmth and comfort and to balance the subtle energy bodies. It can be connected to energize the root chakra and harnessed to heal the sacral.

Citrine also aids confidence through its link to the solar plexus. Personal power, intuition, and higher wisdom can all be developed by working with this gemstone as can emotions and any emotional issues in the sacral. Although it is primarily for the solar plexus and sacral it can also be used to enhance spiritual qualities relating to the crown chakra.

Citrine brings confidence, self-expression, and releases stresses and tensions. The digestive and nervous systems can be balanced with citrine, and emotions, wounds, and traumas can be gently released and healed.

Crystal Personality: Confident, happy, and sunny. You enjoy expressing yourself creatively and exploring the subtle realms of mind and spirit.

Qualities: Warming, comforting, uplifting, and healing. Brings confidence and creative expression.

Chakras: Solar plexus with links to the root, sacral, and crown.

Topaz

Topaz is a golden yellow crystal relating to the solar plexus. It has stabilizing, balancing, and energizing qualities that can be used to direct and focus energy. It helps cleanse emotions or negative energy holding you down. It also inspires confidence and has a stimulating effect.

Topaz can spark personal power, leadership, and confidence whilst simultaneously balancing and clearing any negative emotions or imbalances.

Crystal Personality: People who resonate with this crystal are self-assured and are natural leaders. If channeled positively, you are supportive and can reach a high position in life (negative associations include manipulation and being overly dominant).

Qualities: Energizing, balancing, clearing, and stimulating.

Chakra: solar plexus

Peacock Ore

Peacock ore is a range of colors and is primarily for the solar plexus. It can stimulate all of the main chakras and the subtle energy bodies. Peacock ore's main color is gold and its energy encourages happiness, joy, and self-empowerment. It can create inner contentment and general satisfaction in life.

Peacock ore can also be used to protect you from harm, negativity, and unwanted energies.

Crystal Personality: Enthusiastic and content in life. You may be mature, well-traveled, or have much life experience. You also have an underlying confidence which radiates out.

Qualities: Clearing, harmonizing, integrating, and expanding.

Chakra: solar plexus with links to the crown

Pyrite

Pyrite is also known as fool's gold and is formed by water merging with or coming into contact with extremely hot rocks. Pyrite can be used to strengthen and aid in the healing of the physical body. It is also known to have a gentle cleansing and detoxifying effect on the digestive system due to its iron composition.

Pyrite can also be used to overcome depression, anxiety, and frustration and protect you from pollution and negative energy.

Crystal Personality: Ambiguous, evasive, or misunderstood. You may be a dreamer and highly connected to spiritual ways of perceiving.

Qualities: Soothing, cleansing, clearing, protecting, and healing.

Chakra: solar plexus

Amber

Amber carries the energy of sunlight and brings feelings of warmth, relaxation, and comfort. This crystal also stimulates the mind and is great to connect to for intellectual or educational pursuits.

Amber reflects the beginnings and origin of the earth as it is fossilized resin which formed from pine trees over 50 million years ago. It can stimulate and enhance the nervous system, release anxiety, and calm the mind. It can also be used to alleviate depression, induce feelings of deep peace, and calm an overactive brain.

Crystal personality: Intellectual, aware, intelligent, and busy. You work hard and enjoy mentally stimulating activities.

Qualities: Warming, comforting, stimulating, and enlivening.

Chakras: sacral and solar plexus (predominantly solar plexus).

Brief recap of crystals covered in this section:

ROOT: Obsidian, Hematite, Black Tourmaline, Smoky Quartz, Red Jasper, Bloodstone, and Garnet

SACRAL: Carnelian, Moonstone, Pearl, and Citrine

SOLAR PLEXUS: Tiger's Eye, Citrine, Topaz, Amber, Peacock ore, and Pyrite

Green, Blue, Indigo & Purple Crystals

Emerald

Emerald is a green crystal for the heart chakra. It brings a soothing harmony to all systems of the body and aids in purification and cleansing. Emerald can allow you to access higher states of consciousness and develop greater spiritual awareness whilst simultaneously releasing fears, anxieties, and concerns.

Emerald can aid in meditation and brings the qualities of peace, growth, and abundance. It is expanding, spiritually-stimulating, and energizing to the senses whilst also increasing feelings of love, kindness, and optimism.

Crystal Personality: Friendly, open, loving, and clear-sighted. If you resonate with emerald you have a silent yet powerful confidence and are optimistic and heart-centered.

Qualities: Cleansing, harmonizing, calming, and energizing. Brings loving and harmonious feelings.

Chakra: heart

Jade

Jade is another crystal for the heart. It is a beautiful green like emerald and has a strong balancing and centering effect when connected to. Jade can stabilize emotions and bring awareness of your physical body. It has a gentle grounding effect whilst connecting you strongly to your heart and higher self through the expansion of consciousness.

Jade can develop spiritual awareness and bring wisdom regarding connection to the planet and natural energies. It also aids all healing processes and increases subtle sensitivities.

Crystal personality: Rooted, grounded, and heart-centered. Strong feelings of family with fine-tuned senses and developed intuition.

Qualities: Integrating, intuitive and instinctual and aware.

Chakra: heart

Interesting fact: In Ancient China, Jade was regarded as one of the most valued gemstones for medicinal use. People would use jade to prolong life and strengthen the lungs, heart, and other major organs.

Malachite

Malachite is a light and dark mixed green crystal with powerful healing properties. It can be used as an effective protective stone due to its ability to absorb and transmute harmful energy. It helps withdraw imbalances from the body and can soothe and reduce pains associated with the muscles and inflammation.

Malachite can be used to clear and heal emotions, bring peace and a sense of balance back into one's life, and cleanse the body of toxins and pollutants.

Crystal Personality: Supportive with a healing and soothing energy. You may be a healer, counselor, or therapist and are both grounded and intuitive.

Qualities: Soothing, purifying, detoxifying, and calming. Relieves pain and transmute negative and harmful energy.

Chakra: heart

Tree Moss Agate

Tree moss agate is essentially a clear quartz with green and sometimes brown inclusions. It can sometimes be translucent and relates to the heart. It can align you with your heart chakra, cleanse and balance emotions, and connect you to nature. Feelings of closeness to the natural world increase when working with tree moss agate and expansion, freedom, and spatial awareness often increase.

Tree moss agate can also specifically be used to aid plant growth and help ill or dying plants who may need some healing. This crystal can help you balance the mind, body, and spirit and relieve tension or anxiety through its relation to the natural world.

Crystal Personality: At ease with nature, abundant, and resourceful. You are a free spirit with a love for the natural world and enjoy your freedom. You may be a poet, dreamer, or earth activist.

Qualities: Opening, cleansing, clearing, and harmonizing. Qualities of nature, curiosity, and spaciousness.

Chakra: heart

Aventurine

Aventurine is a green gem with elements of brown-orange. Aventurine forms when quartz crystals melt and recrystallizes near other minerals. This gemstone is very efficient at balancing the heart and can be connected to overcome any feelings of anxiety. It brings calmness, positivity, and cleanses negative energy. It can be used to release emotional pains and traumas gently and can aid in self-confidence and expression.

Aventurine also is a crystal which is effective for meditation, creative expression, enhancing vision and insight, and developing perception.

Crystal personality: Bright, optimistic, emotionally balanced, and clear-sighted. You may be a natural meditator or engage in visualization and creative pursuits.

Qualities: Tranquilizing, clearing, calming, and harmonizing. Brings insight, creativity, enhanced perception, and confidence.

Chakra: heart

Ruby

Ruby is a gemstone of the heart and of the sun. Ruby heals the heart, both energetically and physically. It brings balance, harmony, self-confidence, clarity, and a sense of ease and grace.

Ruby can connect us with the divine and bring feelings of unconditional love and spiritual expansion. It also can aid in life force energy flow.

Crystal Personality: Warm, friendly, open, and loving. You are confident, honest, trustworthy, and sincere and may be a natural leader or wayshower in some way.

Qualities: Encouraging, stimulating, energizing, and balancing.

Chakras: heart, solar plexus, and crown (predominantly heart)

Rhodonite

Rhodonite is a pink crystal of varying degrees and is primarily for the heart. It can help bring balance, stabilize and harmonize emotions, release stress, anxieties, or tension, and calm emotional responses. It can also increase confidence, motivation, and self-expression and help those who engage in mantras and chanting.

Due to its healing effect on both emotions and subtle energy, rhodonite can be used to aid in romantic relationships in addition to friendships and work partnerships.

Crystal Personality: Grounded, passionate, down-to-earth, and charming. You are confident and self-assured once you have found your direction in life.

Qualities: Grounding, harmonizing, balancing, and motivating. Brings compassion and practicality.

Chakra: heart

Rose Quartz

For a detailed account of rose quartz, see the final section of this chapter.

Amazonite

Amazonite is one of the most common minerals within the earth's crust and is a blue-green color. It can be used to bring harmony, balance, and clarity to the heart and throat chakras and strengthens both the heart and communication. It brings calm and focus and stabilizes the nervous system.

Amazonite is effective for all aspects relating to improving communication, memory, and mental and cognitive abilities. It can also stimulate psychic abilities and increase the ability to perceive subtle energy.

Crystal Personality: Intellectual, a good communicator, and inquisitive. You enjoy learning, discovering, and exploring all aspects relating to consciousness and the higher mind.

Qualities: Calming, balancing, and stabilizing. Inquisitive, curious, and mind-orientated.

Chakras: heart and throat

Turquoise

Turquoise is a light blue to blue-green crystal. In ancient times, people used turquoise as an amulet of protection and saw it as a symbol of wealth. It can be used as a protective stone and to enhance communication, expression, and feelings of love and friendship. It stimulates subtle energies of the different bodies and can be used to connect to spirit and psychic phenomena.

Turquoise can protect you from pollutive, harmful, and negative energies whilst strengthening your spirit and higher mind simultaneously.

Crystal personality: Grounded, balanced, and whole. You are most likely a teacher, guide, or wayshower with strong links to spirituality.

Qualities: Strengthening, supporting, stimulating, and protecting.

Chakra: throat

Aquamarine

Aquamarine is a beautiful and calming yet stimulating blue-green. It is the ideal gemstone for communication and creative expression as it has strong psychic and intuitive influences. Aquamarine can be connected to energize the throat chakra, enhance mood, and increase inspiration.

Aquamarine also aids in love and friendship.

Crystal Personality: Supportive, intuitive, talkative, and imaginative. You are full of stories and ideas and may have a developed sense of psychic ability, higher awareness, and artistic visionary.

Qualities: Clearing, purifying, integrating, and energizing. Strong links to spirit, subtle energy and creativity, and the sea.

Chakras: throat

Blue Lace Agate

Blue lace agate is blue and white and is a form of quartz. This crystal can be used to strengthen the throat chakra and bring feelings of peace, calm, and contentment. It also can aid in subtle and gentle detachment to any situation or feeling that is overwhelming, intense, or stressful.

Blue lace agate has a subtle energy which can be used to connect to the spiritual realms. Despite its gentleness, it is also uplifting and can energize communication.

Crystal Personality: Spiritually-oriented, a dreamer, and a good communicator. You are expressive, a good listener, and enjoy spiritual or creative pursuits.

Qualities: Calming, influencing, uplifting, and energizing.

Chakra: throat

Lapis Lazuli

Lapis lazuli is a deep blue crystal with gold and white spots. Lapis lazuli has many profound qualities and was revered by the ancient Egyptians. It is a dream stone, having a powerful effect on dreaming, dream recall and the ability to lucid dream, in addition to aiding in memory, learning, and the storing of wisdom. It can balance and harmonize the throat and third eye/brow chakras and has an uplifting effect on consciousness and higher mind activities.

Lapis lazuli can bring depth, inner stillness, and silence, aid in meditation, and enhance intuition and inspiration. It is known by some as a crystal for prophets due to its strong link to the subtle and spiritual realms.

Crystal Personality: Deep thinker, philosopher, teacher, or student. You possess intuition, sight, and wisdom at an advanced level and have strong links to the spiritual worlds. Due to the connection to truth and knowledge, you may be involved in law or higher learning.

Qualities: Brings truth, wisdom, consciousness, intuition, inspiration, and aids in dreaming, memory, and meditation.

Chakras: throat and brow/third eye (can be used for both)

Sodalite

Sodalite is another gemstone which relates to both the throat and brow/third eye. Sodalite is deep blue with inclusion and veins and can be used to aid in communication. It can balance both thought processes and emotions and be used to connect the throat and brow/third eye.

As with all blue stones, sodalite can aid in meditation, bring feelings of calmness and peace, and help with all forms of expression. It can also be used for contemplation and introspection.

Crystal Personality: Strong communicator, technologically-oriented, and emotionally aloof or reserved. You tend to be in your mind a lot and are more interested in mental exchanges and interests.

Qualities: Calming, clarifying, and balancing. Brings perceptive, communication, and mental exchanges.

Chakras: throat and brow/third eye

Labradorite

Labradorite is a gray blue-green crystal very powerful for bringing transformation. This gemstone can create shifts in vibration and can enhance awareness. It brings protection and a free flow of energy to the chakras and can remove blockages.

Labradorite can dispel negative energy, protect you, and attract new opportunities into your life.

Crystal Personality: Excitement, sudden changes, and new opportunities. You often attract the unexpected into your life and are both grounded and intuitive.

Qualities: Energy shifting, transforming, surprising, and stimulating.

Chakras: All, but specifically the brow/third eye

Azurite

Azurite is a blue/dark blue crystal and is strongly associated with malachite. This is due to azurite eventually changing into malachite if exposed to high levels of water absorption. Azurite is a rare gemstone however it holds a powerful vibration. It can enhance spiritual energy profoundly and has a transformational quality. Azurite can stimulate deep levels of consciousness, increase intuition, enhance communication, and aid in creative and inspirational expression.

Azurite can also breakdown deep tension and stress stored in the body. It increases energy flow and is a good stone for healers or those wishing to develop their own healing skills.

Crystal Personality: You are a healer either by profession or naturally in daily life. You hold a great power to lift situations to higher levels of awareness and may be mysterious, psychic, or enigmatic.

Qualities: Healing, transforming, integrating, expanding, and understanding.

Chakra: brow/third eye

Celestite

Celestite is a sky blue, clear or clear-transparent blue-gray crystal with strong links to the subtle and spiritual realms. It is formed through volcanic activity and has very powerful energies. Celestite can bring a calm, serene, and joyous state in harmony with the subtle elements of reality. It can lift sadness, depression, or anxiety and enhance intuition.

Celestite is a perfect gem for meditation and can develop the third eye/brow and crown chakras. It also has a particularly calming and clearing effect on communication.

Crystal Personality: Dreamy, contemplative, and meditative. You may be in a world of your own and very connected to some unseen spiritual reality.

Qualities: Light, meditative, otherworldly, and spiritual. Dreamy and calming.

Chakras: brow/third eye and crown

Sapphire

Sapphire is violet or violet-blue however can also be white or yellow. This crystal has a calming and stabilizing effect on many systems of the body and can be used to regulate emotions. It aids in relaxing over-activity and tension and can ease the mind. Communication can be improved with sapphire as can personal expression.

Sapphire can be used to connect to the higher mind, personal expression, subtle states of perception, spiritual energies, visionary experiences, and meditative states.

Crystal Personality: Psychic, spiritual, and connecting to subtle realms of existence. You have high observation skills and possess advanced levels of understanding.

Qualities: Spiritually stimulating, enhancing, regulating, and expanding.

Chakras: brow/third eye and crown

Fluorite

Fluorite is a purple gemstone with strong links to the ether. This crystal helps assimilate ideas and information, aids conscious awareness, and brings new levels of creative genius. Ideas, inventions, and imagination all come under fluorite's realm. It can inspire, bring innovation, and stimulate the mind into new ways of thinking. Fluorite is derived from the Latin word 'fleure' which means to flow.

Crystal Personality: You are a designer or inventor. You may be ahead of your time and highly philosophical, intuitive, or a deep thinker.

Qualities: Inventive, innovative, and original. Energy which inspires and stimulates the mind.

Chakra: brow/third eye

Conclusion

Meditation and your interior calm together with the release of negative emotions also helps you to interpret images or information you receive during screening more accurately. This is vital because the emotional response to what you get while screening has a dramatic impact on the screaming session.

Negative emotions and responses can influence the learning and knowledge you obtain when you practice your various screening techniques. The act of screaming and any other form of mental power requires a multi-level energy exchange, including the emotional experience. What you respond to what you interpret affects the process and decides the outcome of the experience.

Screaming for both beginners and experienced mental can be a strong and transformative experience. Regardless of which screening methods you can choose, screening is an excellent way of developing certain kinds of mental capacity. Screening and day-to-day therapy will allow you to develop a much better understanding of your cognitive capacity.

www.ingramcontent.com/pod-product-compliance
Lightning Source LLC
Chambersburg PA
CBHW071840080526
44589CB00012B/1067